JUVENILE HYPERTENSION

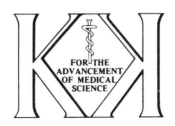
FOR THE ADVANCEMENT OF MEDICAL SCIENCE

Kroc Foundation Series
Volume 8

Juvenile Hypertension

Edited by

Maria I. New, M.D.
Professor and Vice-Chairman,
Department of Pediatrics
Division Head, Pediatric Endocrinology
Director, Pediatric Clinical Research
Center
Cornell University Medical College
New York, New York

Lenore S. Levine, M.D.
Assistant Professor of Pediatrics
Associate Director, Division of
Pediatric Endocrinology
Associate Director, Pediatric Clinical
Research Center
Cornell University Medical College
New York, New York

Raven Press ■ New York

LQM hJ iM

Raven Press, 1140 Avenue of the Americas, New York, New York 10036

Made in the United States of America

International Standard Book Number 0-89004-145-8
Library of Congress Catalog Card Number 76-51556

Preface

This volume, the first devoted to childhood hypertension, is a status report on hypertension in the young. Epidemiology, clinical investigation, experimental work in animal models, hemodynamics, and therapy are considered. The chapters in this book are derived from presentations at a symposium on childhood hypertension held at The Kroc Foundation Ranch in Santa Ynez, California on March 23 to 26, 1976. The invited scientists were asked to concentrate on the special nature of hypertension in children. This resultant volume is not intended as a review of hypertension in general, but rather to bring the reader up to date on the juvenile form of this disease.

The idea that childhood hypertension may be an important health problem is not new. Indeed, the importance of studying childhood hypertension was stressed as early as the Second National Conference on Cardiovascular Diseases held in Washington, D.C. in 1964 (*The Heart and Circulation, Vol. 1, Research,* edited by E. C. Andrus. Federation of American Societies for Experimental Biology. Washington, D.C., 1964). The following statements by some of the leaders in the field of hypertension are quoted from this conference.

> *I. Page, p. 19:* "We must develop the ability to recognize the hypertensive genotype before hypertension develops. Studies of close relatives, especially siblings, of hypertensive patients may have particular usefulness in defining the characteristics of the pre-hypertensive individual. It is clear that the renal-adrenal mechanisms of hypertension require further elucidation so that they may be controlled. While great strides have already been made, the full fruits of this approach have not yet been exploited."
>
> *M. D. Schweitzer and F. R. Gearing, p. 228:* "There is no satisfactory alternative to prospective studies to determine the significance of blood pressure lability in later life, or to measure the comparative risk in children of hypertensives and normotensives. Why is it, then, that there have been so few such studies made?"

Systematic investigation of childhood hypertension is only now beginning to take form and gain importance. Researchers in a number of disciplines are now studying some of the fundamental questions in childhood hypertension including: (1) standards of normal blood pressure, (2) prevalence of hypertension, (3) genetic versus environmental factors in hypertension, (4) regulatory mechanisms of blood pressure, and (5) prognosis and treatment. These are questions that were being asked by investigators of adult hypertension during the period from 1930 to 1945, when active research in arterial hypertension began.

Although some may consider pediatrics equivalent to medicine practiced in midgets, one has only to be faced with the care of children to know that they are not simply small adults. The processes of growth and development strongly affect all clinical observations, including blood pressure. Therefore, hypertension in the young must be studied in the young.

Can we learn lessons from the study of children that are more difficult in adults? Is there extra benefit to the adult in studying hypertension in its earliest stage? Is the study of blood pressure in the child a preventive health measure? I believe the answer is "yes" as illustrated in the following experience: The syndrome of "dexamethasone-suppressible hyperaldosteronism" is associated with high blood pressure in children and in adults. We have just described a new kindred of this disorder involving three children and the mother. Although the childrens' blood pressure decreased promptly with dexamethasone treatment, the mother remained hypertensive. The disorder responds to treatment with dexamethasone in childhood but not in adulthood. Thus, it is necessary to diagnose the syndrome in childhood when hypertension responds to treatment. Failure to do so penalizes the adult patient as well as the child. Further research is required to understand the mechanism of the disorder: why the child responds to treatment and why the adult does not.

Thus, these cases demonstrate the need to investigate hypertension in the child in order to prevent irreversible hypertension in the adult. Hypertension in children is usually free of the associated vascular and neurologic complications observed in adults, and, therefore, hypertension can be studied in children in the "crystalline" state. I believe the child is the best subject for the study of the pathophysiology of hypertension.

There is an excellent exchange of ideas incorporated into the chapters of this book, perhaps the most interesting and stimulating aspect of which is the breaking of barriers between clinicians and experimentalists, both interested in hypertension in the young.

Maria I. New
Editor

Contents

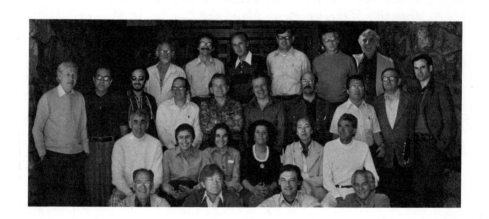

PARTICIPANTS

First Row L to R: Robert L. Kroc, Peter Amacher, Ian Bush, and Kenneth Savard.
Second Row: Bernard L. Mirkin, Jennifer M. H. Loggie, Lenore S. Levine, Maria I. New, Margaret M. Kilcoyne, and Derek A. Denton.
Third Row: Ralph E. Peterson, A. Avinoam Kowarski, Jeremy S. D. Winter, Isidore S. Edelman, Clarence Grim, Jean-Guy Mongeau, Myron Weinberger, Andreas Chrambach, Stanley Ulick, and John P. Rapp.
Fourth Row: Sol Londe, Stephen H. Zinner, Edward G. Biglieri, Ronald Brown, Ron Lauer, and James C. Melby.
Not shown: Harriet P. Dustan.

Contributors

S. K. Anand
Department of Medicine
Specialized Center of Research in
 Hypertension
Indiana University School of Medicine
Indianapolis, Indiana 46202

W. Aoi
Third Department of Medicine
Nagasaki University School of
 Medicine
Nagasaki City, Machi, Japan

Denise Bertrand
Department of Pharmacology
University of Montreal
Montreal, Quebec H3C 3J7, Canada

Edward G. Biglieri
Clinical Study Center
San Francisco General Hospital
and
Department of Medicine
University of California
San Francisco, California 94110

Pierre Biron
Department of Pharmacology
University of Montreal
Montreal, Quebec H3C 3J7, Canada

J. P. Coghlan
Howard Florey Institute of
 Experimental Physiology and
 Medicine
University of Melbourne
Parkville 3052, Australia

Sidney L. Dale
Section of Endocrinology and
 Metabolism
Department of Medicine

Boston University School of Medicine
University Hospital
Boston, Massachusetts 02118

André Davignon
Service of Cardiology
Department of Pediatrics
Sainte-Justine Hospital for Children
Montreal, Quebec H3C 3J7, Canada

D. A. Denton
Howard Florey Institute of
 Experimental Physiology and
 Medicine
University of Melbourne
Parkville 3052, Australia

J. P. Donohue
Department of Medicine and Urology
Specialized Center of Research in
 Hypertension
Indiana University School of Medicine
Indianapolis, Indiana 46202

Harriet P. Dustan
Research Division
Cleveland Clinic
Cleveland, Ohio 44106

Isidore S. Edelman
Cardiovascular Research Institute
University of California School of
 Medicine
San Francisco, California 94143

J. S. K. Fan
Howard Florey Institute of
 Experimental Physiology and
 Medicine
University of Melbourne
Parkville 3052, Australia

David Goldring
Department of Cardiology
Washington University School of
  Medicine
St. Louis, Missouri 63110

Samuel W. Gollub
Edward Mallinckrodt Department of
  Pediatrics
Washington University School of
  Medicine
St. Louis, Missouri 63110

C. E. Grim
Department of Medicine
Specialized Center of Research in
  Hypertension
Indiana University School of Medicine
Indianapolis, Indiana 46202

Antonio Hernandez
Department of Cardiology
Washington University School of
  Medicine
St. Louis, Missouri 63110

Edward H. Kass
Channing Laboratory
Department of Medicine
Harvard Medical School
Boston City Hospital
Boston, Massachusetts 02118

Margaret M. Kilcoyne
Department of Medicine
College of Physicians and Surgeons
Columbia University
New York, New York 10032

A. Avinoam Kowarski
The Harriet Lane Service
Children's Medical and Surgical Center
Johns Hopkins University School of
  Medicine
Baltimore, Maryland 21205

Lenore S. Levine
Department of Pediatrics

The New York Hospital–Cornell
  Medical Center
New York, New York 10021

Jennifer M. H. Loggie
Department of Pediatrics
University of Cincinnati
and
Division of Clinical Pharmacology
The Children's Hospital Research
  Foundation
Cincinnati, Ohio 45229

Sol Londe
Department of Cardiology
Washington University School of
  Medicine
St. Louis, Missouri 63110
and
Pediatrics Department
St. Louis Labor Health Institute
St. Louis, Missouri 63103

Harry S. Margolius
Departments of Pharmacology and
  Medicine
The Medical University of South
  Carolina
Charleston, South Carolina 29401

Anthony L. McCall
Section of Endocrinology and
  Metabolism
Department of Medicine
Boston University School of Medicine
University Hospital
Boston, Massachusetts 02118

J. G. McDougall
Howard Florey Institute of
  Experimental Physiology and
  Medicine
University of Melbourne
Parkville 3052, Australia

John K. McKenzie
Department of Medicine
Nephrology Section

Health Sciences Center
University of Manitoba
Winnipeg, Manitoba R3E 0Z3, Canada

James C. Melby
Section of Endocrinology and
    Metabolism
Department of Medicine
Boston University School of Medicine
University Hospital
Boston, Massachusetts 02118

Claude J. Migeon
The Harriet Lane Service
Children's Medical and Surgical Center
Johns Hopkins University School of
    Medicine
Baltimore, Maryland 21205

Bernard L. Mirkin
Departments of Pediatrics and
    Pharmacology
Division of Clinical Pharmacology
University of Minnesota
Health Sciences Center
Minneapolis, Minnesota 55455

Jean-Guy Mongeau
Department of Pediatrics
Service of Nephrology
Sainte-Justine Hospital for Children
Montreal, Quebec H3T 1C5, Canada
and
Department of Pharmacology
University of Montreal
Montreal, Quebec H3C 3J7, Canada

Maria I. New
Department of Pediatrics
The New York Hospital–Cornell
    Medical Center
New York, New York 10021

Maurice Payot
Service of Cardiology
Albert Calvette Hospital
59000 Lille, France

Lourdes M. Pichardo
Department of Pediatrics
Service of Nephrology
Sainte-Justine Hospital for Children
Montreal, Quebec H3T 1C5, Canada

Leyla C. Ramirez
Veterans Administration Hospital
Bronx, New York 10468

John P. Rapp
Department of Medicine
Medical College of Ohio
Toledo, Ohio 43614

Christian Rey
Department of Pediatrics
Service of Cardiology
Sainte-Justine Hospital for Children
Montreal, Quebec H3T 1C5, Canada

Bernard R. Rosner
Channing Laboratory
Department of Medicine
Harvard Medical School
Boston City Hospital
Boston, Massachusetts 02118

B. A. Scoggins
Howard Florey Institute of
    Experimental Physiology and
    Medicine
University of Melbourne
Parkville 3052, Australia

Alan Sinaiko
Department of Pediatrics and
    Pharmacology
Division of Clinical Pharmacology
University of Minnesota
Health Sciences Center
Minneapolis, Minnesota 55455

Robert C. Tarazi
Research Division
The Cleveland Clinic
Cleveland, Ohio 44106

Stanley Ulick
Veterans Administration Hospital
Bronx, New York 10468

Myron H. Weinberger
Department of Medicine
Specialized Center of Research in
  Hypertension

Indiana University School of Medicine
Indianapolis, Indiana 46202

Jeremy S. D. Winter
Department of Pediatrics
Endocrinology Section
Health Sciences Center
University of Manitoba
Winnipeg, Manitoba R3E 0Z3, Canada

Juvenile Hypertension, edited by
M. I. New and L. S. Levine. Raven
Press, New York © 1977.

Prevalence of Hypertension and Distribution of Causes

Jennifer M. H. Loggie

*Department of Pediatrics, University of Cincinnati, Cincinnati, Ohio 45229; and
Division of Clinical Pharmacology, The Children's Hospital Research Foundation,
Cincinnati, Ohio 45229*

The subject of this chapter is the epidemiology of hypertension and the distribution of its causes in the young. It is my intention to summarize what has been published about the incidence and prevalence of hypertension in young people and to describe what is presently known about the etiology of hypertension in children and teenagers.

Since the early 1970s, interest in childhood hypertension has escalated and attention is now at last focusing on whether those individuals with essential hypertension in adult life can be identified in adolescence or even childhood. In 1971, Londe et al. (13) and I (11) published separate papers in which we independently suggested that the entity euphemistically known as "essential hypertension" might have its origins in early life and that a better understanding of its etiology and pathogenesis might be obtained by studying children rather than adults with fixed hypertension. In the same year, Zinner et al. (22) published their observations indicating that there is a familial aggregation of blood pressure in children.

INCIDENCE

The actual incidence of hypertension in children and adolescents is not yet known. The data in Table 1 indicate that approximately 1 to 11% of children and adolescents have high blood pressure. My question remains: What actually constitutes "hypertension" at various ages? Table 1 includes results from 13 screening studies on young populations published during the last 20 years. Interpretation of the data presented is difficult for a variety of reasons. First, different investigators have used different definitions for identifying young hypertensives. In addition, in some studies subjects are supine, in

1

TABLE 1. *Prevalence of hypertension in people under 30 years of age*[a]

Author (yr published)	Country of study	Position in which BP taken	Definition of hypertension or borderline hypertension (mm Hg)	Incidence (%) of hypertension found, sex	Total no. of patients screened	Age range (yr)	Total no. of males and females in group	Race
Boynton and Todd (1947)	USA (MN)	Sitting	SBP > 140 DBP > 90	7.36, M 1.12, F 5.87, M 2.18, F	72,210	16–30	42,382 M 29,828 F	Not stated specifically
Masland et al. (1956)	USA (MD)	Not stated	BP > 140/90	1.4, (17 M, 8 F)	1,795	Adolescents	Not stated	Not stated specifically
Heyden et al. (1969)	USA (GA)	Sitting	Average of 3 readings: SBP > 140 or DBP > 90	11	435	15–25	219 M 216 F	186 Black; 249 white
Londe (1966)	USA (MS)	Supine Supine	Labile: BP > 90th percentile, 1 reading Persistent–repeated BP > 95th percentile	12.4, M 11.6, F 1.9 (14 M, 21 F)	1,805 1,805	4–15 4–15	894 M 911 F 894 M 911 F	92 Black; 1,713 white 92 Black; 1,713 white
Wilber et al. (1972)	USA (GA)	Sitting	SBP > 160 (1st reading) DBP > 95 (1st reading)	1 1.5	799	15–25	Not stated	799 Black
Kotchen et al. (1974)	USA (DC)	Sitting	SBP > 140	10, Black M 1, Black F	797	17–20	Not stated	Predominantly black
Kilcoyne et al. (1974)	USA (NY)	Sitting Sitting	SBP ≧ 140 DBP ≧ 90 SBP ≧ 140 DBP ≧ 90	SBP 5.4 DBP 7.8 SBP 1.2 DBP 2.4	First screen: 3,537 Rescreen of hypertensives: 215 of 277 from 1st screen	14–19	Not stated	2,193 Black; 124 white; 1,220 Latin

Study	Location	Position	Criteria	Prevalence (%)	No. screened	Age (yr)	Sex/No.	Population
Lauer et al. (1975)	USA (IA)	Sitting	SBP ≥ 140 DBP ≥ 90	SBP 8.9 DBP 12.2 Both-SBP and DBP 4.4 / SBP 4.9 DBP 8.2	1,301 / 3,528	14–18 / 6–13	Not stated	4,829 subjects (6–18 yr screened once): 96.4% white; 0.6% black; 2.8% Spanish American; 0.1% Oriental; 0.1% American Indian
Reichman et al. (1975)	USA (NY)	Sitting Left arm	SBP ≥ 140 DBP ≥ 90	5.9 2.5	1,863 Rescreen of hypertensives: 46	12–20 (90% 14–17)	Not stated	1,449 Black; 388 white; 26 other
Johnson et al. (1975)	USA (GA)	Sitting	SBP ≥ 140 DBP ≥ 90	20.5 (3 readings—1st used for statistical analysis)	546	15–29	Not stated	326 Black; 220 white
Bøe et al. (1957)	Norway	Sitting	BP 150–160/90–95	1.04, F 3.01, M	3,833	15–19	1,532 M 2,301 F	Norwegian
Mathewson et al. (1965)	Canada	Not stated	SBP 140–159	10.8	1,957	15–29	All M	North American
Kimura and Ota (1965)	Japan	Not stated	SBP ≥ 160 and/or DBP ≥ 95 (if BP less than 140/90, considered normotensive.)	0.6 (9.2, borderline)	2,728	0–19	1,255 M 1,473 F	Japanese

BP, blood pressure; SBP, systolic blood pressure; DBP, diastolic blood pressure; M, male; F, female.
aSee also Weiss et al., ref. 20
Results from 10 studies in U.S. and 3 in other countries.

others sitting, and in yet others, position is unspecified. Different instrumentation has been used; in some studies, the diastolic blood pressure has been determined by the fourth Korotkoff sound, whereas in others the disappearance of sounds (5th Korotkoff) has been taken to represent diastolic pressure. Not all authors have broken down the prevalence of hypertension in their population by age, sex, and race; in addition, it is difficult to ascertain the length of time that subjects had been in a given position before blood pressure was measured. And these are just some of the problems.

It should also be noted that most of the studies reported are cross-sectional and that rescreening of those identified initially as "hypertensive" has infrequently been reported. Kilcoyne et al. (6) and Reichman et al. (18), who reported rescreening in New York City, found that significantly fewer "hypertensives" remained "hypertensive" at a second examination. This is also our impression from rescreening patients referred to us by local clinics and pediatricians. Furthermore, second, third, and fourth blood pressure measurements in our clinic are often lower than readings at a first visit.

It is well known that the proper cuff size for measuring blood pressure in children and teenagers is important, and the cuff size is not always specified by the investigators reporting screening studies. This is relevant, particularly because in some investigations there has been a positive correlation between hypertension and obesity. Finally, detailed data on the socioeconomic status of the study populations are given infrequently, and the time of year when the blood pressure measurements were made is not always recorded.

DEFINITIONS

I would like now to concentrate on definitions of hypertension in youngsters, if one can, in fact, specify what constitutes abnormal blood pressure at any given age. To define what is abnormal, one must depend on published values for normal blood pressure at various ages, and this again is difficult. For many years, I have depended on Londe's 1966 data (12); although they are cross-sectional, I consider them valuable because blood pressure was measured in an office situation. For want of a better definition (and lacking long-term follow-up studies, I have reservations about it), we and others have considered children and teenagers at possible high risk for the later development of sustained hypertension if their systolic and/or diastolic blood pressure has frequently been ≥ 90th percentile for age. Currently, we are actively tracking ± 100 such individuals but we have not yet reached any firm conclusions since the longest follow-up of this "borderline" group is only 5 to 6 years. Nomenclature also presents a problem in the published literature; for example, I hedge by calling these individuals "possibly borderline hypertensives," whereas Londe and his co-workers (13), in their paper published in 1971, call their patients "hypertensive" if they had had systolic and/or diastolic blood pressure ≥ 90th percentile for 1 year.

Again, most of the published data on the normal distribution of blood pressure in youngsters, except those of McCammon (16), have been obtained from cross-sectional studies; this is a self-evident problem inasmuch as we do not yet know whether children and teenagers continue to track at the same blood pressure level with time. Although McCammon's data are longitudinal, it must be borne in mind that the children he followed were highly selected and that his population is therefore not representative of the general population in the United States. In addition, one should not accept norms established between 1927 to 1967, because some investigators have found a change in blood pressure distribution on restudying this question only 10 years since that time in the same locality.

Londe's data for males and females were presented separately and seemed to differ somewhat between sexes, particularly during puberty. On the other hand, the data of Lauer et al. (9) were not broken down by sex, because, I believe, these investigators found no significant differences between the sexes. Londe's subjects were supine and his population was predominantly white. The subjects of Lauer et al. were sitting and almost 100% of their population was also white. Voors (19), from New Orleans, recently presented a paper suggesting that blacks by the age of 10, and possibly earlier, have higher blood pressures than whites. Reichman et al. (18) also found that black males had higher blood pressure than black females who, in turn, had higher blood pressure than white females. Their sample of white males was too small to analyze with significance. These authors also found a higher incidence of hypertension in the black high school students they studied as compared to the whites.

I recently saw a composite figure of the mean blood pressures of children and teenagers of various ages from several studies performed in the United States, and the differences were quite striking. For example, the mean blood pressures of children in the Bogalusa, Louisiana heart study (1) were remarkably lower than those from any other study and, in particular, because they were temporally related, from those obtained in the study of Lauer et al. in Muscatine, Iowa (9). One wonders whether these differences are due simply to differences in methodology or whether there is a real geographical difference in the distribution of blood pressure. I feel an answer to this is important, particularly since the Muscatine population was almost entirely white and the Bogalusa population, a mixture of both black and white, included a higher risk ethnic group.

I mentioned the importance of different positions when blood pressure is measured. The effect that changes in posture may have on blood pressure is shown in Fig. 1. This is a fairly common finding in patients with "borderline hypertension" (11). Because changes in blood pressure can occur with changes in position, it appears invalid to take data from several studies in which pressure has been measured in different positions and using different techniques and to combine these data in order to arrive at a *normal* distribution curve. Apparently, this was done recently by Mitchell et al. (17).

It is to be hoped that within the next 10 years or so, longitudinal sex, race,

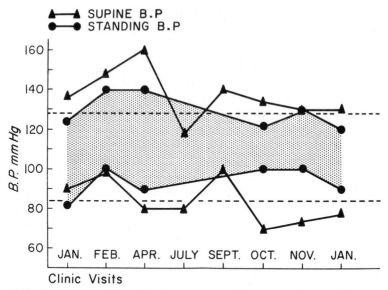

FIG. 1. Differences in supine and standing blood pressure in a child followed for border-line hypertension. The dotted lines represent the 95th percentile for systolic and diastolic pressure.

and age-specific follow-up data on blood pressure distribution in children and adolescents will be available because some studies of this nature are already underway. After traveling around the country during the past 2 to 3 years, visiting programs that have ongoing or proposed epidemiological studies involving blood pressure measurements in children and adolescents, I have been recurrently and forcibly struck by the different methodologies already in use or proposed for use. It seems to me that, individuality in research aside, it would be both helpful and more economical to use standardized protocols for both screening and tracking in various parts of the country. I will illustrate the present problem. In Cincinnati, the Lipid Research Center has used the random-zero muddler for measuring early morning blood pressure in a school-age population. In Bogalusa, under as near to basal conditions as it is possible to achieve in the field, both the physiometrics instrument and mercury sphygmomanometers have been used. In Muscatine, Lauer's group measured blood pressure in the afternoon, also using mercury sphygmomanometers.

One should question the effect that all of these variables have on the data finally generated. The results of epidemiological studies as presently structured obviously can cause confusion for the practicing physicians who must rely on them for guidance.

ETIOLOGY OF HYPERTENSION

I now present a discussion of the etiology of hypertension in youngsters. In 1969 (10), I wrote that "essential hypertension" was uncommon in this population, and subsequent studies from other medical referral centers seem to bear out this impression. In 1971, Londe and associates (13) published their findings on asymptomatic "hypertensive" children found to have elevated blood pressure on routine office physical examination. They found that the vast majority of their patients had no definable underlying cause for hypertension. Presumably, the discrepancy between the findings of Londe et al. and those reported by others at that time was due in large part to (a) the unselected nature of their population, (b) the fact that diagnostic evaluations were performed in patients with lower blood pressure levels than were being evaluated elsewhere, and (c) the fact that rather attenuated diagnostic evaluations were often performed. In reports from other medical centers, children and adolescents were being studied for hypertension rather extensively only when their supine diastolic blood pressure was persistently > 90 mm Hg.

In the last 6 years, my patient population has been expanded to include the type of patient reported by Londe et al. (13), that is, asymptomatic youngsters identified on routine physical examination in the offices of local pediatricians as having "borderline hypertension." Most of these patients are now simply followed clinically. Those with supine diastolic blood pressure persistently ≥ 90 mm Hg, whom we have called "definite hypertensives," have had diagnostic evaluations; by 1974 to 1975, we had concluded that 55% of our patients, aged 12 to 18 years, had primary, idiopathic, or essential, hypertension. Figure 2 summarizes some of the published studies regarding the incidence of primary and secondary hypertension in the young.

Our population remains somewhat skewed, however, because I do not see, except for therapeutic reasons, patients with coarctation of the thoracic aorta or those with the chronic glomerulonephritides. Skewed as our population is, however, our figures do suggest that essential hypertension occurs with some frequency before the age of 20. Even though our youngest patient with this diagnosis was 3 years old at the time of initial evaluation, essential hypertension in our experience is less common in the very young than in adolescents. Similarly, within our adolescent group, we have frequently found an underlying cause for hypertension in white females and relatively few in this race–sex class have had primary hypertension.

We no longer perform an extended diagnostic evaluation, trying to rule out all of the known causes of hypertension in youngsters with elevated blood pressure. Based on accumulated negative data with studies of the adrenal hormones (Table 2), we now perform these measurements only when they are indicated on clinical grounds. We long ago came to regard the history, family history, and physical examination to be of paramount importance in directing the laboratory and X-ray studies ordered for young hypertensives.

Figure 3 shows our yield of positive and negative intravenous pyelograms and abdominal angiograms in hypertensive patients aged 2 to 12 years and those aged 12 to 20 years as of mid-1974. Thirty-six of the pyelograms were performed by the rapid-sequence technique, 25 by the regular technique, and for 5, done elsewhere and reported to us, the sequence was not specified.

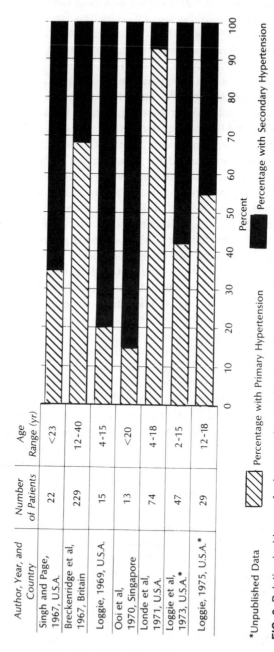

Author, Year, and Country	Number of Patients	Age Range (yr)
Singh and Page, 1967, U.S.A.	22	<23
Breckenridge et al, 1967, Britain	229	12-40
Loggie, 1969, U.S.A.	15	4-15
Ooi et al, 1970, Singapore	13	<20
Londe et al, 1971, U.S.A.	74	4-18
Loggie et al, 1973, U.S.A.*	47	2-15
Loggie, 1975, U.S.A.*	29	12-18

Percentage with Primary Hypertension

Percentage with Secondary Hypertension

*Unpublished Data

FIG. 2. Relative incidence of primary and secondary hypertension in the young, reported in six different studies, is depicted.

TABLE 2. *Adrenal studies in 67 patients, aged 2 to 20 years, presenting with diastolic blood pressure ≥ 90 mm Hg*

Adrenal hormones measured	Total	Normal	Abnormal
Urine 17-OHS, 17-KS, and/or plasma cortisols	29	26	3[a]
Aldosterone secretion rates or plasma aldosterone	32	30	2
Urinary catecholamines and VMA	46	41	5[b]

17-OHS, 17-hydroxysteroid; 17-KS, 17-ketosteroid; VMA, vanillylmandelic acid.

[a]One patient on birth control pills.
[b]Four diagnostic of neural crest tumors.

Table 3 summarizes the diagnosis of 75 young patients evaluated by me for hypertension in my institution and is self-explanatory.

Our experience with the diagnostic evaluation of young borderline hypertensives is now more extensive than that summarized in Table 4, which, again, covers the period up to mid-1974. All have had urinalyses, most have had chemistries (including electrolytes, blood urea nitrogen, creatinine, and uric

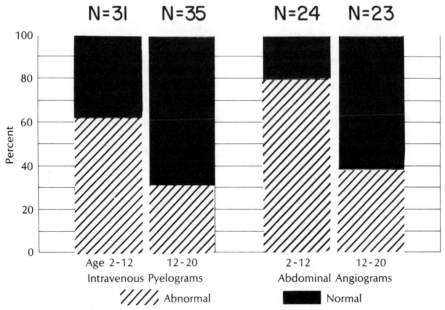

FIG. 3. Intravenous pyelography and abdominal angiography have yielded more abnormal findings in patients aged 2 to 20 years. Whereas specific diagnostic studies to detect an underlying cause of hypertension are frequently productive in younger children, the yield is significantly lower among adolescents, confirming that primary hypertension is relatively common in the latter.

TABLE 3. *Causes of sustained hypertension (supine DBT >
90 mm Hg) in 75 patients < 20 years of age*[a]

Idiopathic without any disease other than obesity	29 (13)
Idiopathic with associated diseases of questionable relationship to hypertension	10
Bilateral pyelonephritis/dysplastic kidney	13
Unilateral renal parenchymal disease	8
Renal artery stenosis	5
Catecholamine-producing tumors	4
Other tumors	3
Abdominal coarctation/hypoplastic aorta	2
Renal parenchymal disease not considered pyelonephritic	1

[a]Excludes all transient forms of hypertension, thoracic coarctation, and glomerulonephritides.

TABLE 4. *Studies in 41 patients, aged 12 to 18 years, presenting with borderline hypertension*

Tests performed	Total	Normal	Abnormal
Intravenous pyelogram	20	20	0[a]
Urine 17-OHS, 17-KS, and/or plasma cortisols	8	8	0
Aldosterone secretion rates or plasma aldosterone	6	6	0
Urinary catecholamines and VMA	20	20	0

17-OHS, 17-hydroxysteroid; 17-KS, 17-ketosteroid; VMA, vanillylmandelic acid.

[a]Fourteen fast-sequence and four regular intravenous pyelograms were performed. In two cases, the second sequence was not recorded.

TABLE 5. *Diagnoses in borderline hypertensives with underlying organic disease*

Diagnoses	Race	Sex	Age (yr)
Diffuse arteriopathy	Black	Male	5
Caliectasis left kidney	White	Female	5
Intrarenal cysts	Black	Female	16
Unilateral hydronephrosis	Black	Male	5
Unilateral dysplastic kidney	White	Female	9
Neuroblastoma	Black	Female	8
Hypothyroidism and goiter	Black	Maie	20
Hypothyroidism and goiter	Black	Female	19

acid), and many have had electrocardiograms and chest X-rays, as well as the studies noted in the table. We have had a low yield of laboratory and X-ray abnormalities in these patients; however, in Table 5, I have listed the organic underlying diseases detected in this group. In every case, there was some clinical observation that suggested the need for further diagnostic evaluation. In other words, clearly not all young patients with what I call "borderline hypertension" have idiopathic hypertension and some, on clinical grounds, demand an extended evaluation.

REFERENCES

1. Berenson, G. (1976): Louisiana State University. *Personal communication.*
2. Bøe, J., Humerfelt, S., and Wedervang, F. (1957): The blood pressure in a population: Blood pressure readings and height and weight determinations in the adult population of the city of Bergen. *Acta Med. Scand.* [*Supp.*], 321:1.
3. Boynton, R. E., and Todd, R. L. (1947): Blood pressure readings of 75,258 university students. *Arch. Intern. Med.,* 80:454.
4. Heyden, S., Bartel, A. G., Hames, C. G., and McDonough, J. R. (1969): Elevated blood pressure levels in adolescents, Evans County, Georgia. *JAMA,* 209:1683.
5. Johnson, A. L., Carnoni, J. C., Cassell, J. C., Tyroler, H. A., Heyden, S., and Hames, C. G. (1975): Influence of race, sex and weight on blood pressure behavior in young adults. *Am. J. Cardiol.,* 35:523.
6. Kilcoyne, M. M., Richter, R. W., and Alsup, P. A. (1974): Adolescent hypertension. I. Detection and prevalence. *Circulation,* 50:758.
7. Kimura, T., and Ota, M. (1965): Epidemiologic study of hypertension. Comparative results of hypertensive surveys in two areas in Northern Japan. *Am. J. Clin. Nutr.,* 17:381.
8. Kotchen, J. M., Kotchen, T. A., Schwertman, N. C., and Kuller, L. H. (1974): Blood pressure distribution of urban adolescents. *Am. J. Epidemiol.,* 99:315.
9. Lauer, R. M., Connor, W. E., Leaverton, P. E., Reiter, M. A., and Clarke, M. S. (1975): Coronary heart disease risk factors in school children. The Muscatine Study. *J. Pediatr.,* 86:697.
10. Loggie, J. M. H. (1969): Hypertension in children and adolescents. I. Causes and diagnostic studies. *J. Pediatr.,* 74:331.
11. Loggie, J. M. H. (1971): Systemic hypertension in children and adolescents: Causes and treatment. *Pediatr. Clin. North Am.,* 18:1273.
12. Londe, S. (1966): Blood pressure in children as determined under office conditions. *Clin. Pediatr.,* 5:71.
13. Londe, S., Bourgoignie, J. J., Robson, A. M., and Goldring, D. (1971): Hypertension in apparently normal children *J. Pediatr.,* 78:569.
14. Masland, R. P., Jr., Heald, F. P., Goodale, W. T., and Gallagher, J. R. (1956): Hypertensive vascular disease in adolescence. *N. Engl. J. Med.,* 255:894.
15. Mathewson, F. A., Brereton, C. C., Keltie, W. A., and Paul, G. I. (1965): The University of Manitoba follow-up study: A prospective investigation of cardiovascular disease. II. Build, blood pressure and electrocardiographic factors possibly associated with the development of coronary heart disease. *Can. Med. Assoc. J.,* 92:1002.
16. McCammon, R. W. (ed.) (1970): Vital signs—blood pressure and pulse. In: *Human Growth and Development.* Charles C Thomas, Springfield, Ill.
17. Mitchell, S. C., Blount, S. G., Jr., Blumenthal, S., Hoffman, J. I. E., Jesse, M. J., Lauer, R. M., and Weidman, W. H. (1975): The pediatrician and hypertension. *Pediatrics,* 56(1):3.
18. Reichman, L. B., Cooper, B. M., Blumenthal, S., Block, G., O'Hare, D., Chaves, A. D., Alderman, M. H., Deming, Q. B., Farber, S. J., and Thomson, G. E. (1975): Hypertension testing among high school students. I. Surveillance procedures and results. *J. Chronic Dis.,* 28:161.

19. Voors, A. W., Foster, T. A., Frerichs, R. R., and Berenson, G. S. (1975): Some determinants of blood pressure in children age 5–14 years in a total biracial community—the Bogalusa study. Presented at the Annual Meeting of the American Heart Association, Anaheim, Calif.
20. Weiss, N. S., Hamill, P. V. V., and Drizd, J. (1973): Blood pressure levels in children 6–11 years: Relationship to age, sex, race and socioeconomic status. US DHEW Publication (HRA) 74-1617. Vital and health statistics data from the National Health Survey, Series 11, No. 135, pp. 1–24.
21. Wilber, J. A., Millward, D., Baldwin, A., Capron, B., Silverman, D., James, L. M., Wolbert, T., and McCombs, N. J. (1972): Atlanta community high blood pressure. Methods of community hypertension screening. *Circ. Res.,* 31(Suppl. II):101.
22. Zinner, S. H., Levy, P. S., and Kass, E. H. (1971): Familial aggregation of blood pressure in childhood. *N. Engl. J. Med.,* 284:401.

Juvenile Hypertension, edited by
M. I. New and L. S. Levine. Raven
Press, New York © 1977.

Blood Pressure and Hypertension in Children: Studies, Problems, and Perspectives

*,†Sol Londe, *David Goldring, **Samuel W. Gollub, and *Antonio Hernandez

*Department of Cardiology, and **Edward Mallinckrodt Department of Pediatrics, Washington University School of Medicine, St. Louis, Missouri 63110; and †Pediatrics Department, St. Louis Labor Health Institute, St. Louis, Missouri 63103*

STUDIES

There is increasing evidence in recent years that primary hypertension is much more prevalent in children than was previously conceived. This is most apparent when blood pressure determination is part of the routine physical examination in pediatric practice. Because more physicians are now measuring blood pressure in their young patients, a critical evaluation of the definition of juvenile hypertension is essential. This was the first problem when our studies began about 16 years ago. The frequently mentioned arbitrary value of 130/85 to 140/85–90 mm Hg for juvenile hypertension did not seem appropriate for children of every age (1–11). Also, the data on blood pressure measurements from studies of population samples of normal children (12–19) (Fig. 1) varied considerably because of the different methodology used by the investigators. Thus, it was decided to establish normal standards for office practice.

The means, standard deviations, 90th and 95th percentiles for each age and sex were calculated for 795 boys and 798 girls, 3 to 15 years of age (20,21) (Figs. 2 and 3). Readings were recorded in a standardized manner; that is, the pressures were obtained in the right arm in supine well children at the end of routine physical examinations. Cuffs of the appropriate width for arm length and the mercury manometer were employed. The fifth Korotkoff phase was considered to be the diastolic endpoint, and one reading was used unless the pressure seemed high, in which case the lowest of three readings was employed. These values have served as our guidelines.

We have followed the suggestion by Master et al. (22) for the adult population that pressures persistently above the 90th percentile are considered to be suspicious, and those above the 95th percentile to be hypertensive. Thus,

13

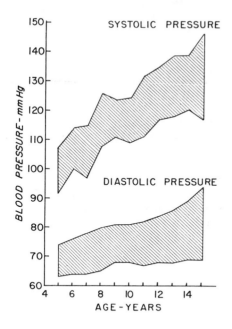

FIG. 1. Ranges for 95th percentiles for systolic and diastolic pressures found in the literature. (From Londe, ref. 20.)

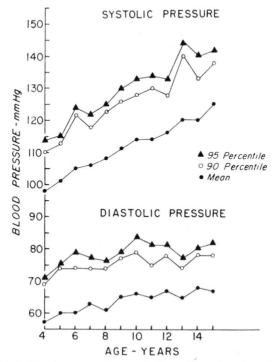

FIG. 2. Blood pressure for age in boys. (From Londe, ref. 20.)

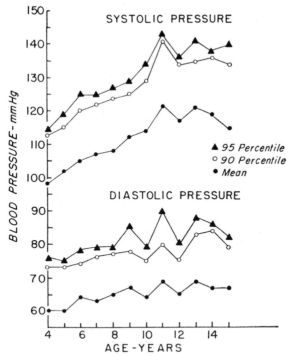

FIG. 3. Blood pressure for age in girls. (From Londe, ref. 20.)

patients in our office are considered hypertensive if their systolic and/or diastolic pressures remain repeatedly above the 90th percentile, and occasionally above the 95th percentile for 1 year or more.

To date, 132 such patients have been followed for 2 to 9 years. Hypertension was found as early as 3 years of age and in 29 children before the age of 6 (Fig. 4). The largest number of hypertensive readings was recorded at ages 5 and 8 to 12 years. Forty-one percent had systolic, 42% systolic and diastolic, and 17% diastolic hypertension. Thirty percent had normal pressure before they became hypertensive (Table 1). One-half of 98 patients with three or more readings had an occasional normal reading suggesting that they had labile hypertension. Sixty-five percent of 81 children observed from 3 to 9 years still had elevated pressure at their last examination. Fifty-one percent had a parent or parents with hypertension and 5% of the families had more than one hypertensive child. Obesity was present in 55%. The incidence of parental hypertension in normotensive children was 18%, and 15% were obese.

The first 74 hypertensive children, 4 to 18 years of age, were reported in 1971 (23). Initially, 33 subjects were investigated on an outpatient basis and had the following laboratory investigations: serum sodium and potassium levels, urea clearance, 24-hr urinary catecholamine excretion, electrocardi-

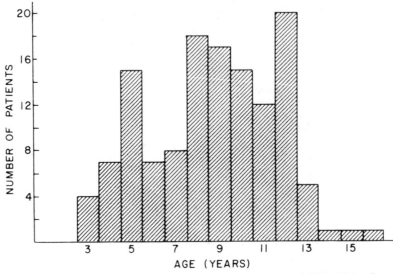

FIG. 4. Age at which hypertension was first documented (131 children).

ogram, chest roentgenogram, and intravenous pyelogram when indicated. Because of the paucity of findings in this group, more extensive inpatient investigations were done on the next 41 patients in the clinical research unit of St. Louis Children's Hospital. Laboratory examinations included serum sodium, potassium, chloride, creatinine, urea nitrogen, and plasma renin activity. The latter was done after the children had been ambulatory for 30 to 60 min. Twenty-four-hour urinary excretion of aldosterone, sodium, creatinine, and creatinine clearance was determined. In addition, catecholamines were measured in two urine specimens obtained on successive days, and

TABLE 1. *Findings in 132 hypertensive children*

Findings	Percent
Systolic hypertension	41
Systolic and diastolic hypertension	42
Diastolic hypertension	17
Normal pressure documented before appearance of hypertension	30
One-half of 98 patients with 3 or more readings had labile hypertension	
Parental hypertension	51
Overweight	55
Families with more than 1 hypertensive child	5
Sixty-five percent of 81 patients, followed for 3–9 years, had elevated pressures at their last examination	
Possible etiology all related to urinary tract	5
Primary hypertension	95

rapid-sequence intravenous pyelograms, chest roentgenograms, and electro-cardiograms were performed. Thirty-nine normotensive children, 4 to 14 years of age, also received the same inpatient examination excepting catecholamine determination, intravenous pyelogram, chest roentgenogram, and electro-cardiogram.

With one exception, our last 58 patients have had outpatient investigation. Thirty-two have had creatinine clearance, serum potassium, creatinine, and urea nitrogen determination, rapid-scan intravenous pyelograms, chest roent-genograms, and electrocardiograms. Rapid-scan intravenous pyelogram was performed in only 1 of the remaining 25 subjects.

A possible cause for hypertension was found in only 5%. All had disease of the urinary tract, that is, one patient with decreased maximum urea clearance and elevated nonprotein nitrogen, one with ureteral reflux, one with renal bleeding associated with sickle-cell trait, and three with pyelonephritis. Thus, 95% of children in whom high blood pressure was an incidental finding seemed to have primary hypertension. Because of our experience, we do not think that extensive investigations are necessary in the absence of suspicious history, symptoms, or findings.

Although the observations described indicate that the suggested definition of juvenile hypertension is a useful one, there is still considerable hesitancy concerning its acceptance. The ultimate answer will be found when we examine those of our patients who are now young adults. However, several facts indicate that the concept is probably valid: first is the significantly high incidence of parental hypertension and of obesity; second, 60% of 48 patients considered to be hypertensive before the age of 10 had blood pressure readings $\geq$ 140 systolic and/or 90 mm Hg diastolic at one time or another.

Additional epidemiological studies in our center have considered blood pressure in black and white children 3 to 14 years of age, and in students of five high schools in the metropolitan St. Louis area. In the latter investigation, which is still in progress, the question of standards, incidence of high blood pressure, and possible differences in blood pressure in black and white adolescents are also being examined.

In the first investigation, blood pressure measurements were made in 585 black and 566 white girls, and in 710 black and 620 white boys (3 to 14 years of age). All of the black children were patients in an inner city health center with the exception of 198 who, along with all of the white subjects, were clients of a prepaid union health center. Blood pressure measurements were made by one physician in the city clinic and another in the union health center. The method previously described was used, except that the fourth Korotkoff sound served as the diastolic pressure value.

The findings were surprising when the mean pressures in the two races were compared. The mean systolic pressures in the black children were either lower or not significantly different in 92% of the 12 age groups (Figs. 5 and 6). The same was true for diastolic pressure in 88% of the age samples. Elevated

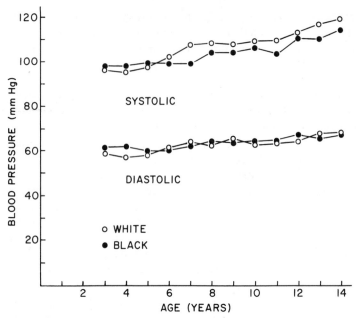

FIG. 5. Mean systolic and diastolic blood pressures in 710 black and 620 white boys (3 to 14 years of age).

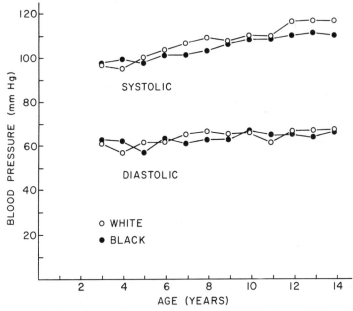

FIG. 6. Mean systolic and diastolic blood pressures in 585 black and 566 white girls (3 to 14 years of age).

systolic readings, that is, pressures above the 90th percentile for age and sex, were found in 2.2% of the black children and 1.85% of the white children; this difference was not significant. Since the disappearance of the sounds was used for our diastolic standard, we did not investigate the incidence of diastolic hypertension. Since systolic pressure correlated with weight in this population sample, the mean weights of the children in the two races were compared. The mean weights were not significantly different in 88% of the age groups for both boys and girls.

In the high school study, 2,050 black and 4,808 white children (14 to 18 years of age) were screened. Pressures were taken in the seated position by specially trained senior student nurses. The fifth Korotkoff phase was used for the diastolic signal, and the average of the last two of three readings was used for analysis.

The blood pressures of the girls were significantly lower than those of the boys except for the ages 14 and 15 (Fig. 7). In the latter age groups, the diastolic pressures of the girls were higher. The values were similar in the 16- to 18-year age group of the boys and in all of the female groups. Using the mean + 1.65 SD as the level for suspect hypertension, and the mean + 2 SD as hypertension, the following standards were suggested (Table 2): for the boys, 133/82 to 138/86 for age 14, 137/85 to 141/89 for age 15, and 140/87 to 144/91 for ages 16 to 18; for the girls, 128/83 to 132/87 for ages 14 to 18.

At initial examination, 466 students (6.8% of the total) had pressures above the 90th percentile (mean + 1.65 SD) and were checked on three other occasions by the project physicians. Persistent hypertension was found in 175 (2.5%) who were invited to come into St. Louis Children's Hospital for investigation. Only 1 of 81 children examined, a girl with exophthalmic goiter, had a finding related to hypertension.

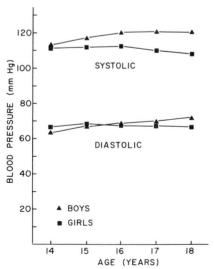

FIG. 7. Mean systolic and diastolic blood pressures in 3,494 males and 3,364 females (14 to 18 years of age).

TABLE 2. *Suggested upper limits of normal blood pressure*[a] *for children 14 to 18 years of age*

Subjects	Age (yr)	Suspicious level mm Hg (mean + 1.65 SD)	Hypertensive level mm Hg (mean + 2 SD
Boys	14	133/82	138/86
	15	137/85	141/89
	16–18	140/87	144/91
Girls	14–18	128/83	132/87

[a]Taken in seated position, average of second and third readings.

Comparison of blood pressures in the black and white students showed the same pattern observed in the younger children (Figs. 8 and 9). Both systolic and diastolic pressures were significantly higher in the white males. There was no significant difference in the systolic pressures of the black and white girls, but the diastolic pressures were higher in the white. The incidence of initial pressures above the 90th percentile was 8% for the white and 6.7% for the black students.

Thus, our findings indicate that the tendency toward higher incidence of hypertension in our adult black population does not begin during the first two decades of life. Finally, the concept accepted by many clinicians that a high-blood pressure is a normal physiologic phenomenon during puberty was examined in 418 boys and girls 10 to 14 years of age. The possible relationship between blood pressure and serum follicle stimulating hormone, luteinizing hormone, stage of breast development, menarche, and duration since menarche in girls and stage of pubic hair development in boys was investigated. There was no significant correlation with any of these criteria of sexual

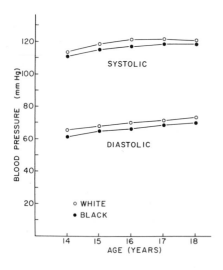

FIG. 8. Mean systolic and diastolic blood pressures in 992 black and 2,502 white males (14 to 18 years of age).

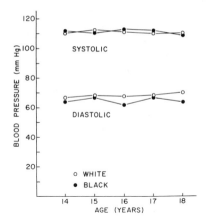

FIG. 9. Mean systolic and diastolic blood pressures in 1,058 black and 2,306 white females (14 to 18 years of age).

maturation and we have concluded that high blood pressure during puberty should be viewed with suspicion.

PROBLEMS

(a) Foremost, is the establishment of blood pressure standards and a generally accepted definition of hypertension in the young. A uniform methodology, taking into consideration position, cuff size, one reading or multiple readings, and diastolic signal, is needed to resolve this problem.

(b) Are there regional differences as has been suggested, and if so, can one set of standards be used universally?

(c) Do blood pressures in population samples change with time? Our first data were collected in the late 1950s and early 1960s, whereas the last two studies were done in the early 1970s. In the racial study on the 3- to 14-year-old children, the mean systolic pressures were lower in 10 of the white male-age groups than in the first investigation, which was on predominantly white children (Figs. 10 and 11). Seven of the differences were significant. This was also true for the girls except that the differences were significant in only three age samples. Since different diastolic signals were used, diastolic pressure was not compared. Similarly, in the study on blood pressure and puberty, both systolic and diastolic pressure were significantly lower in both sexes.

(d) Are we justified in doing a minimum work-up on asymptomatic children in whom hypertension is an incidental finding?

(e) Should the patients we have described be treated with nonpharmacologic means such as weight reduction of the obese, avoidance of excessive salt intake, or regular exercise regimen?

(f) Pending investigation of the possible effects of the antihypertensive drugs on growth and development, is drug treatment justified? If so, at what level of hypertension should therapy be started? There is still no general agreement about when to start treatment of the adult hypertensive.

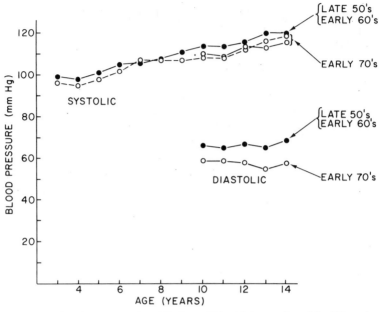

FIG. 10. Mean blood pressures in white boys (3 to 14 years of age) in different years.

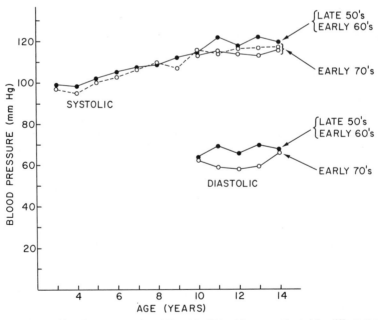

FIG. 11. Mean blood pressures in white girls (3 to 14 years of age) in different years.

(g) Are we too drug oriented in treating the disease?

(h) Should systolic hypertension be disregarded despite evidence that it, too, has an effect on longevity and plays a role in the development of complications? (24,25)

PERSPECTIVES

Two interesting areas of investigation are suggested by the recent blood pressure studies in children. First, is the long-term study of hypertensive children into adult life. We hope to be able to do this in the first group of children we have reported, many of whom are now young adults. Second, is the exciting prospect of studying the disease in its early stages by mass screening of the young and at its inception by regular examinations of the siblings of hypertensive children, and of the offspring of hypertensive parents.

ACKNOWLEDGMENTS

This work was aided in part by grants from the St. Louis and American Heart Associations and contributions from The Arthur United Fund and the Alpha Phi Sorority, St. Louis Chapter.

REFERENCES

1. Daeschner, C. W., Jr. (1960): Evaluation of the child with arterial hypertension. *J. Miss. State Med. Assoc.,* 1:535.
2. Haggerty, R. J., Maroney, M. W., and Nadas, A. S. (1956): Essential hypertension in infancy and childhood. *Am. J. Dis. Child.,* 92:535.
3. Slater, R. J., Geiger, D. W., Azzopardi, P., and Webb, B. W. (1959): Hypertension in children. *Can. Med. Assoc. J.,* 81:71.
4. McRory, W. W., and Noonan, J. A. (1960): Hypertension in childhood. *J. Iowa Med. Soc.,* 50:188.
5. Oliver, W. J., Talner, N. S., and Stern, A. M. (1960): Hypertension in infancy and childhood. *J. Mich. Med. Soc.,* 59:82.
6. Meilman, E., Kurtz, M., and Turner, L. B. (1961): Hypertension in childhood. *J. Mt. Sinai Hosp.,* 28:196.
7. Rosenheim, M. C. (1961): Hypertension in children. *Proc. R. Soc. Med.,* 54:1093.
8. Katcher, A. L. (1964): Hypertension in adolescent children. *Med. Clin. North Am.,* 49:1467.
9. Losse, H. (1966): Behandlung der Juvenilin Hypertonie. *Dtsch. Med. Wochenschr.,* 91:2130.
10. Page, L. B. (1966): Childhood hypertension. Etiology, investigation and treatment. *Mass. Gen. Hosp. Rounds Clin. Pediatr.,* 5:39.
11. Loggie, J. M. H. (1969): Hypertension in children and adolescents. I. Causes and diagnostic studies. *J. Pediatr.,* 74:331.
12. Stocks, P., and Karn, M. W. (1924): *Blood Pressure in Early Life—A Statistical Study.* Cambridge Press, London.
13. Faber, H. K., and James, C. (1921): Blood pressures in children. Clinical application of statistical methods to the interpretation of deviation from the normal average. *Am. J. Dis. Child.,* 22:7.
14. Richey, H. G. (1931): The blood pressure in boys and girls before and after puberty. *Am. J. Dis. Child.,* 42:1281.
15. Shock, N. W. (1944): Basal blood pressure and pulse rate in adolescents. *Am. J. Dis. Child.,* 68:16.

16. Schwenk, A., Eggers-Hahmann, G., and Gensch, F. (1955): Artieller Blutdruck Vasomotorismus und Menarcheteim bei madchen im 2 Lebensjahrzehnt. *Arch. Kinderheilk.,* 150:235.
17. Hahn, L. (1952): The relation of blood pressure to weight, height and body surface area in school boys age 11 to 15 years. *Arch. Dis. Child.,* 27:43.
18. Johnson, B. C., Epstein, F. H., and Kjelsberg, M. O. (1965): Distribution and familial studies of blood pressure and serum cholesterol levels in a total community. Tecumseh, Michigan. *J. Chronic Dis.,* 18:147.
19. Graham, A. W., Hines, E. A., Jr., and Gage, R. P. (1945): Blood pressure in children between the ages of 5 and 16 years. *Am. J. Dis. Child.,* 69:203.
20. Londe, S. (1966): Blood pressure in children as determined under office conditions. *Clin. Pediatr.,* 5:71.
21. Londe, S. (1968): Blood pressure standards for normal children as determined under office conditions. *Clin. Pediatr.,* 7:400.
22. Master, A. M., Dublin, L., and Marks, H. (1950): The normal blood pressure range and its clinical implications. *JAMA,* 143:1464.
23. Londe, S., Bourgoignie, J. J., Robson, A. M., and Goldring, D. (1971): Hypertension in apparently normal children. *J. Pediatr.,* 78:569.
24. Gubner, R. S. (1962): Systolic hypertension. A pathologic entity. *Am. J. Cardiol.,* 9:773.
25. Kannel, W. B., Castell, W. P., McNamara, P. M., McKee, P. A., and Feinleib, M. (1972): Role of blood pressure in the development of congestive heart failure. *N. Engl. J. Med.,* 287:781.

Juvenile Hypertension, edited by
M. I. New and L. S. Levine. Raven
Press, New York © 1977.

Adolescent Hypertension

Margaret M. Kilcoyne

*Department of Medicine, College of Physicians and Surgeons, Columbia University,
New York, New York 10032*

The finding of a 30% prevalence of hypertension in males and 35% in females in the 21- to 55-year age group among 4,220 adults in the Harlem community raised the question as to the age of onset of hypertension in the black population (4). Consequently, two high schools were chosen for blood pressure screening and the following methodology was employed: a standard mercury manometer was used, blood pressure cuffs were selected to cover approximately two-thirds of the upper arm, and the first and fifth Korotkoff sounds were taken as the systolic and diastolic blood pressures, respectively. When the sounds could be heard throughout, the fourth Korotkoff sound was recorded over zero. After 5 min of quiet rest, blood pressure was measured in the left arm with the subject seated; two measurements were taken and the second value was used for statistical purposes. The arbitrary criterion used for an elevated pressure was 140/90 mm Hg. Blood pressures were measured by community health workers who had been trained in our program for 6 months.

The frequency distribution of blood pressure in 3,537 black, Latin, and white high school students revealed four characteristics of blood pressure behavior in this age group (5). Figure 1 depicts the frequency distribution of diastolic blood pressure in males and indicates the lower range of pressures in adolescents compared to adults. The range is similar in all racial groups; however, the proportion of white males in the sample is significantly smaller than the others so that this comparability needs further confirmation in a balanced population sample. An additional difference is the lower systolic blood pressures of females compared to males at this age. These three characteristics point to the need for selecting criteria for abnormal blood pressure levels on the basis of normal adolescent patterns rather than according to adult standards.

The fourth characteristic, to which I will allude again in subsequent confirmatory data, is the added dynamism of the cardiovascular system owing to growth and maturation, which must be considered in evaluating this basically

25

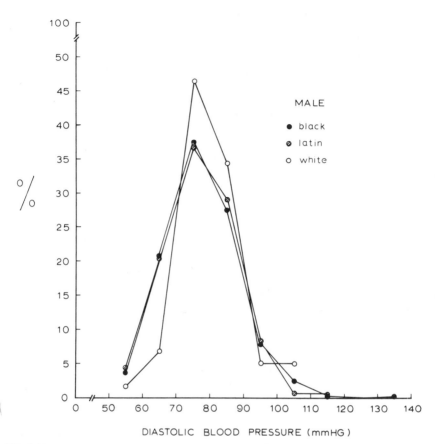

FIG. 1. Frequency distribution curves show the percent of male adolescents with diastolic blood pressures occurring within each 10-mm Hg increment of pressure. No racial difference is observed within the normal distribution. In adolescence, the frequency distribution extends over a lower range of pressures than in adulthood and females have lower systolic pressures than males of the same age group. (From Kilcoyne et al., ref. 5, with permission.)

dynamic system. Figure 2 illustrates the sequential diastolic blood pressure curves in males at ages 14, 16, and 18 years. With progressive maturation, the range of blood pressures increases to higher levels until at 18 years when the rightward skewing, usually seen in adult frequency distribution curves, is apparent. This striking shift is not as apparent in female adolescents, but there is a suggestion that it may occur earlier. The evidence that the basal blood pressure is in a state of flux at this age suggests that repeated measurements may be required to determine the pressure profile of individual adolescents.

The means of the systolic and diastolic blood pressures are given in Table 1 and a comparison is provided with levels obtained in two other studies of 15- to 24-year-old subjects (1,8). The systolic blood pressures among blacks are

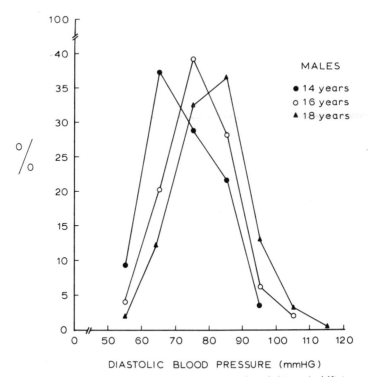

FIG. 2. Frequency distribution curves show a progressive rightward shift toward adult blood pressure ranges observed at ages 14, 16, and 18 years in male adolescents. (From Kilcoyne et al., ref. 5, with permission.)

higher in these studies compared to our data, whereas the diastolic pressures are comparable. The difference in systolic pressure cannot be fully explained by the differences in sample size, proportion of black and white subjects, or geographic location because a comparable influence should have been exerted on diastolic pressure means. From these data, our current working criteria for observation of blood pressures in adolescents include two categories: (a) Those with sustained blood pressures equal to or greater than the mean plus 2 SD (males: 145/95 mm Hg; females: 135/90 mm Hg) are considered as possible hypertensive individuals. (b) Those with blood pressures between 1 and 2 SD above the mean are receiving observation only (males: 132/85 mm Hg; females: 123/82 mm Hg). Whether adolescents stratify at a given level and how or whether this is related to the development of hypertension remains to be determined.

According to our previous criteria of 140/90 mm Hg in both sexes, an overall prevalence of 5.4% systolic and 7.8% diastolic hypertension was obtained on initial screening of this adolescent population. Ten days later, rescreening revealed a marked decline in prevalence to 1.2% systolic and 2.4% diastolic hypertension. In the literature, prevalence figures of from <1 to >34% have

TABLE 1. *Comparison of blood pressure means in adolescents*

Group	Muskegee County, Georgia[a] 15–24 yr (mm Hg)	(n)	Evans County, Georgia[b] 15–24 yr (mm Hg)	(n)	New York, New York 14–19 yr (mm Hg)	(n)
	Systolic blood pressure					
White males	123 ± 9	(44)	127 ± 13	(112)	121 ± 13	(57)
Black males	126 ± 15	(37)	129 ± 14	(77)	118 ± 13	(942)
Latin males	—		—		118 ± 15	(516)
White females	113 ± 11	(56)	120 ± 11	(106)	110 ± 11	(67)
Black females	126 ± 19	(37)	125 ± 14	(82)	112 ± 13	(1,251)
Latin females	—		—		111 ± 12	(704)
	Diastolic blood pressure					
White males	74 ± 10	(44)	75 ± 11	(112)	76 ± 9	(57)
Black males	78 ± 10	(37)	75 ± 9	(77)	74 ± 11	(942)
Latin males	—		—		74 ± 10	(516)
White females	66 ± 12	(56)	79 ± 13	(106)	71 ± 9	(67)
Black females	78 ± 15	(37)	79 ± 10	(82)	72 ± 10	(1,251)
Latin females	—		—		72 ± 10	(704)

The first value given is the mean ± standard deviation. (n) Denotes the number studied.

The means of the diastolic blood pressures in 3,537 black, Latin, and white adolescents reveal no racial differences and are comparable to those published in the two other studies. Systolic blood pressure means are lower in females than in males and are also lower in blacks than observed in the other studies.

[a]Reference 1.
[b]Reference 8.
(From Kilcoyne et al., ref. 5, with permission.)

been reported (3,11). However, these reports were made on the basis of one or two measurements just as those of our previous data, and the validity of these may be questioned on the basis of the degree of blood pressure variability that is apparent during the adolescent years.

Black males had a persistently higher prevalence of hypertension (3.5%) than others in the study group; consequently, a further analysis by age was made (Fig. 3). Black and Latin females show only a slight rise in the prevalence of hypertension in each age group from 14 to 19 years. This contrasts with the pattern in black males who show a sharp rise in the prevalence rate of systolic hypertension from 6.4% at 17 years to 14.5% at 18 years and from 11.7 to 17.3% diastolic hypertension during the same period; Latin males also show this trend. The confluence of factors that may be responsible for this apparent increase in hypertension during the adolescence of black and Latin males is unknown. However, such an early emergence of hypertension in a group that is particularly vulnerable in the adult population deserves further study as well as confirmation.

Subsequent to these initial studies, the question of blood pressure instability in adolescents was investigated by serial measurements over the course of 1 year. Following an initial blood pressure screening of 817 students at a high

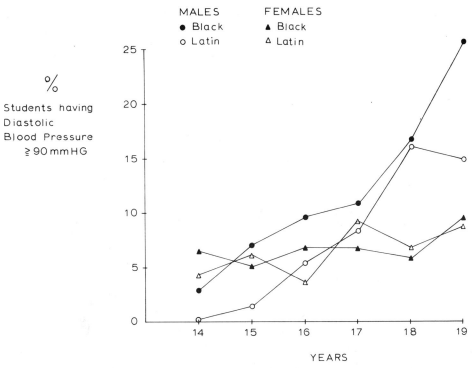

FIG. 3. The percent of students with elevated blood pressure levels is shown sequentially between the ages of 14 and 19 years. A striking increase in the prevalence of hypertension is evident in black and Latin males between 17 and 18 years of age. (From Kilcoyne et al., ref. 5, with permission.)

school health fair, four to six blood pressures were measured by two physicians in three groups of students. Group 1 consisted of all those with systolic or diastolic blood pressures at the 2-SD level or higher; Group 2 consisted of all those with pressures between the levels of 1 and 2 SD above the previously established means in the school. Group 3 was composed of students matched for age, sex, and race with Groups 1 and 2. These adolescents had initial blood pressures less than 1 SD above the mean. The preliminary results for Groups 1 and 2 are shown in Table 2. The intraclass correlation (10) was used to compare the variability of serial blood pressure measurements within each individual with the variability of the serial measurements among the individual students. In this analysis, the initial blood pressure reading was omitted. There was no significant correlation between serial readings in either Groups 1 or 2, indicating that a high degree of variability was present. When the initial blood pressure level was compared with the mean of all subsequent measurements, the correlation was low, verifying the high level of variability among sequential blood pressures in the same adolescents. One exception was noted in the diastolic pressure readings of males in Group 1; when these data were

TABLE 2. *Serial blood pressure measurements in adolescents*

Blood pressure	Intraclass correlation		Correlation coefficient	
	Group 1	Group 2	Group 1	Group 2
Males	(n = 17)	(n = 22)	(n = 17)	(n = 22)
Systolic	0.26	0.30	0.06	0.46
Diastolic	0.30	0.20	0.62[a]	0.25
Females	(n = 15)	(n = 19)	(n = 15)	(n = 19)
Systolic	0.31	0.52	0.19	0.28
Diastolic	0.24	0.51	0.40	0.48
	ns[b]	ns	ns	ns

The left-hand column shows the *r* values for the intraclass correlation between serial blood pressure measurements within a single individual and compared to other adolescents. The right-hand column displays the correlation coefficient between the initial blood pressure level during school screening and the mean of all subsequent readings. The high degree of variability from one blood pressure measurement to the next in a series is indicated by a correlation that is statistically not significant. One value that was significant at the 1% level was attributable to one individual.

[a]$p < 0.01$

[b]ns, Not statistically significant.

plotted, it became apparent that one individual with a single blood pressure elevation accounted for the apparently significant correlation. The *r* value fell to 0.22 when this individual was omitted. The frequency distribution of the standard deviations of the serial blood pressure measurements was uneven and showed a rightward skewness, confirming, in still another way, the difficulty of obtaining a blood pressure profile of individual adolescents after up to six measurements. These findings underscore the uncertainty of prevalence figures for adolescent hypertension based on an isolated measurement and the need for circumspection before labeling an individual adolescent as having hypertensive disease.

Some adolescents do, however, manifest sustained elevations of blood pressure that warrant diagnostic evaluation. Of 27 adolescents who were admitted from the original study in 1972, 17 had persistent levels of diastolic blood pressure at or higher than 2 SD above the mean for their sex and age group (6). No specific etiology could be found for the observed hypertension in any one of these patients; consequently, a diagnosis of primary or essential hypertension was made by exclusion. Plasma renin activity was determined by the radioimmunoassay of angiotension I, and the results in adolescents were compared to those of 146 adult hypertensive patients in the same community (7). Plasma renin activity was normal in 36%, low in 39%, and high in 25% of adult patients in relation to the concomitant urinary sodium excretion. Of the adolescent hypertensive patients, nine had normal, three had low and four had high plasma renin activity (Fig. 4). Ten of these patients whose diastolic blood pressures averaged 105 mm Hg were entered into the same treatment protocol as that established for adult patients (Table 3). Stage I of

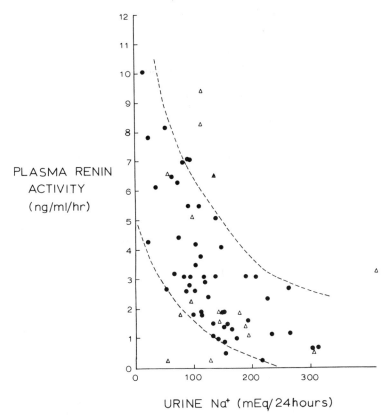

FIG. 4. Plasma renin activity, as determined by the radioimmunoassay of angiotensin I, is plotted against the concomitant urinary sodium excretion in normal subjects and in adolescents with essential hypertension. Δ, Adolescents with essential hypertension; •, normal subjects; (---), range of normal subjects. (From Kilcoyne, ref. 6, with permission.)

the protocol consisted of diuretic therapy for 4 weeks; 48% of adult patients in all renin groups responded with satisfactory control, averaging a 20-mm Hg decline of diastolic pressure. An additional 27% of patients were controlled under Stage II of the protocol in which α-methyldopa (Aldomet®) was added to the diuretic. Thus, 75% of adults with long-standing hypertension of a mean diastolic level of 111 ± 14 mm Hg were well controlled on this regimen. The results in adolescents contrasted sharply (Fig. 5). Satisfactory control in these otherwise healthy adolescents was arbitrarily set at a level below 1 SD above the mean for the age and sex group. This level was not achieved by any patient on the Stage I diuretic protocol. One patient who was initially treated with 300 mg spironolactone did reach this level but was equally well controlled with 80 mg propranolol. When the diuretic alone failed to reduce the blood pressure to optimal levels, α-methyldopa was added; however, this regimen was success-ful in only one of four patients. At this point, the development of gynecomas-

TABLE 3. *Treatment protocol for adult patients*

	Treatment protocol		Response (All renin groups)	Renin group Low = 57% Normal = 40% High = 38%
I.	Spironolactone or	(50–100 mg)		
	Chlorthalidone (Creatine > 2mg%)	(100 mg)	48%	
II.	Spironolactone plus	(50–100 mg)		
	α-Methyldopa	(up to 2g)	26%	
III.	Spironolactone plus	(50–100 mg)		
	Guanethidine	(up to 600 mg)	8%	
IV.	Hydralazine plus III		8%	
	Other: salt restriction only spironolactone 300 mg failure to take medications		18%	

Diuretic therapy (Stage I treatment protocol) effected satisfactory blood pressure control in nearly half the adult hypertensive patients in the Harlem community. This response contrasts sharply with that observed in adolescent hypertensive patients under the same protocol.

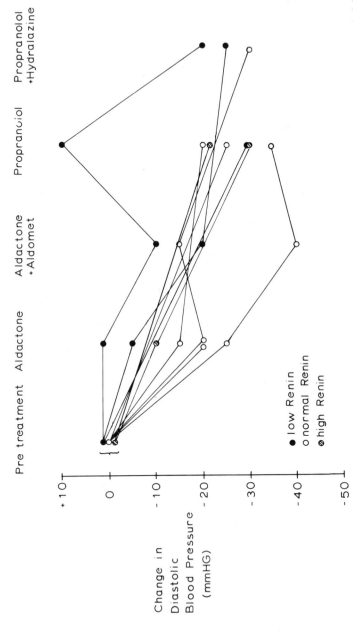

FIG. 5. Response to treatment in relation to the plasma renin activity is depicted as the change in mm Hg from control level. Adolescent hypertensive patients failed to achieve optimal blood pressure control (≤ mean + 1 SD) on diuretic therapy but responded satisfactorily to propranolol or propranolol plus hydralazine. (From Kilcoyne, ref. 6, with permission.)

tia in two adolescent males and the concern as to the possible influence spironolactone might have on adrenal mechanisms in the maturing physiology led to discontinuance of the protocol and initiation of treatment with propranolol. Within 10 days, six students were controlled optimally with propranolol (40 to 120 mg/day) and three more, all with diastolic pressures greater than 110 mm Hg, were controlled following the addition of hydralazine. One of these latter patients had low plasma renin activity, and a paradoxical rise in both blood pressure and renin level occurred during propranolol therapy; the addition of hydralazine brought the blood pressure to desired levels and plasma renin activity returned to pretreatment levels. The reasons for the dichotomy in therapeutic results in adolescents compared to adults remain speculative. This may be merely a skewed sample with results compounded by small size but there is the possibility that this could relate to the physiology of early hypertension. Some of these findings are in accord with those reported in early adult hypertension (2) and in the spontaneously hypertensive rat (9).

In summary, the blood pressure range in a large, predominantly black and Latin, adolescent population has been described and criteria established for possible hypertension in relation to these data. One striking finding, most pronounced in males, is the sequential shift of the entire frequency distribution of blood pressure toward adult levels between 14 and 18 years of age. This factor adds a further increment of dynamism to an inherently dynamic system and suggests that basal blood pressures may be difficult to ascertain in this age group. This was borne out by the high degree of variability observed in serial blood pressure measurements during the course of 1 year. The low correlation between readings indicates that an isolated measurement has little capacity to define the blood pressure profile of an adolescent or to provide a prognosis for future blood pressure behavior in individual adolescents.

REFERENCES

1. Comstock, G. W. (1957): An epidemiologic study of blood pressure levels in a bi-racial community in the southeastern United States. *Am. J. Hyg.,* 65:271–283.
2. Frohlich, E. D., Kozal, V. J., Tarazi, R. C., and Dustan, H. P. (1970): Physiological comparison of labile and essential hypertension. *Cir. Res.,* 26 and 27(Suppl. 1):1–55 and 1–69.
3. Johnson, A. L., Cornoni, J. C., Cassel, J. C., Tynoler, H. A., Heyden, S., and Hames, C. G. (1975): Influence of race, sex and weight on blood pressure behavior in young adults. *Am. J. Cardiol.,* 35:523–530.
4. Kilcoyne, M. M. (1973): Hypertension and heart disease in the urban community. *Bull. N.Y. Acad. Med.,* 49:501–509.
5. Kilcoyne, M. M., Richter, R. W., and Alsup, P. (1974): Adolescent hypertension. I. Detection and prevalence. *Circulation,* 50:758–764.
6. Kilcoyne, M. M. (1974): Adolescent hypertension. II. Characteristics and response to treatment. *Circulation,* 50:1014–1019.
7. Kilcoyne, M. M., Thomson, G. E., Branche, G., Williams, M., Garnier, C., Chiles, B., and Soland, T. (1974): Characteristics of hypertension in the black population. *Circulation,* 50:1006–1013.

8. McDonough, J. R., Garrison, G. E., and Hames, C. G. (1964): Blood pressure and hypertensive disease among Negroes and whites. A study in Evans County, Georgia. *Ann. Intern. Med.,* 61:208–213.
9. Nagaoka, A., Kikuchi, K., and Anamaki, Y. (1969): Depressor responses of the spontaneously hypertensive rats to the anti-hypertensive agents. *Jap. J. Pharmacol.,* 19:401–408.
10. Snedecor, G. W. (1956): *Statistical Methods.* Iowa State College Press, Ames, Ia.
11. Vital and Health Statistics (1964): *Data from the National Health Survey.* Blood pressure of adults by race and area 1960–1962. Public Health Service Publication No. 1000-Series II, No. 5.

Juvenile Hypertension, edited by
M. I. New and L. S. Levine. Raven
Press, New York © 1977.

Comment: Hypertension in Childhood— Magnitude and Nature of the Problem

Lenore S. Levine

It is evident that several factors complicate the determination of the magnitude of juvenile hypertension: first, the lack of a generally accepted definition of hypertension in the young; second, determination of the best way to measure blood pressure in childhood; and third, the lack of knowledge concerning the significance of labile versus sustained hypertension and the number of blood pressures taken to determine hypertension. Long-term follow-up of children with labile hypertension and tracking of children in different percentiles is necessary to provide the answers. What evaluation should be undertaken on the hypertensive child? The younger the child, the more symptomatic the child, the more severe the hypertension, the more thorough the evaluation should be.

The need for establishing the proper criteria for hypertension was demonstrated by New et al.,[1] who presented data on the blood pressure variation in adolescents with mild essential hypertension. Using the criteria for hypertension of 140/90, many adolescents whose blood pressure was greater than the 90th percentile for age would not be included in the suspect group. In addition, New's studies suggested that the lability of blood pressure in childhood and adolescents is less than that observed in adults.

---

[1]New, M. I., Baum, C. J., and Levine, L. S. (1976): Nomograms relating aldosterone excretion to urinary sodium and potassium in the pediatric population: Their application to the study of childhood hypertension. *Am. J. Cardiol.,* 37:658–666.

Juvenile Hypertension, edited by
M. I. New and L. S. Levine. Raven
Press, New York © 1977.

Familial Aggregation of Blood Pressure and Body Weight

*,**Jean-Guy Mongeau, **Pierre Biron, and **Denise Bertrand

*Department of Pediatrics, Service of Nephrology and Pediatric Research Department, Sainte-Justine Hospital for Children, Montreal, Quebec H3T 1C5; and **Department of Pharmacology, University of Montreal, Montreal, Quebec H3C 3J7, Canada*

The Montreal Adoption Survey was undertaken in 1972 as a cross-sectional study of French Canadian families of the Montreal area. Each family had at least one adopted child of the same ethnic origin; the study was done with the purpose of discriminating between the genetic and the environmental components of the familial resemblance of cardiovascular risk factors, such as systolic and diastolic blood pressure, pulse rate, body weight, and weight/height ratio. Natural children, living in these adoptive homes, served as controls.

The study, covering a 2-year period between 1972 and 1974, included 398 families with at least one adopted child. An examination was performed by a nurse during a home visit on 558 adopted and 256 natural children (aged 1 to 20), as well as 356 fathers and 398 mothers. The children included 420 boys and 389 girls.

Families with a relatively recently adopted child (aged 1 year or more) were easier to trace by the adoption agency and these parents were more likely to accept the nurse's visit. Consequently, our population of adopted children shows a preponderance of adoptees below the age of 10 (Fig. 1). This distribution was not comparable to that of the natural siblings whose ages were more evenly distributed, and a bias was thus introduced; that is, the duration of exposure to family customs was longer for our population of natural children. Later in the presentation, we will return to this aspect of our survey.

The nurse visited the family at home in the evening; the family members were examined in a random order. The blood pressure was taken in a sitting position and two readings were averaged to yield a single value for both the systolic and the diastolic. A midparental score was obtained by averaging the

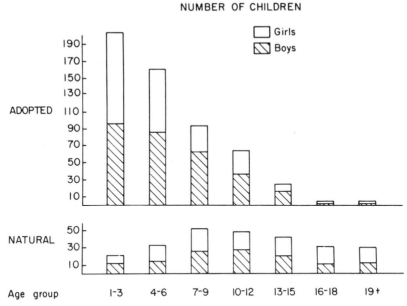

FIG. 1. Population of children examined.

father's and mother's score for each family. In order to make only one comparison per family, one child was randomly chosen as an index case in families with more than one child of the same status, and this applied to natural as well as to adopted children.

Millimeters of mercury were converted into age- and sex-adjusted standard deviation unit scores, where a unit is a reading of an individual minus the mean pressure for his age and sex group over the standard deviation for that group. Three-year age groups were formed for children and 10-year groups for parents.

The mean blood pressure of adopted children did not differ from that of natural children within each age group, a finding in line with the identity of the racial background and living area.

To estimate aggregation, the Pearson coefficient r was computed, using the score of each natural child against the mean score of his natural parents and the score of each adopted child against the mean score of his adoptive parents. In addition, the determination coefficient $r^2 \times 100$ was used. This coefficient describes the percentage of association between the child's score and that of his parents. In the case of blood pressure, this coefficient expresses the percentage variation of the child's blood pressure caused by the blood pressure of his parents.

Child–child correlations were also calculated by choosing a pair of children in the 80 homes with more than one natural child and in the 138 homes with more than one adopted child.

RESULTS

The median values curve of the French Canadian children did not differ from that reported by Moss and Adams (2). It is, however, approximately 10 mm of mercury lower than the blood pressure curve of American children according to data published in 1973 by the United States Department of Health (1). Such a difference could be explained by the fact that in our study, the blood pressure was taken at home when the child was more relaxed; in addition, the French Canadian child is smaller in size than the American child. Several studies have reported a certain correlation between adolescents' blood pressure and their body size.

The median curve of the parents' blood pressure was also not different from the normal values for North American Caucasians.

The resemblance between the parents and children is shown in Fig. 2. There is a very highly significant positive correlation between the blood pressure of

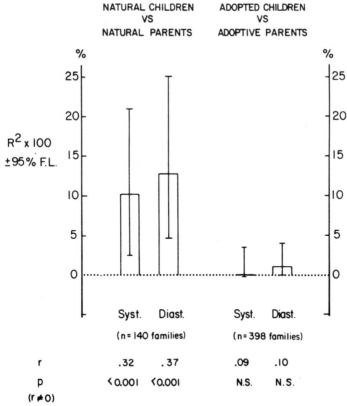

FIG. 2. Determination coefficients in percentage for natural and adopted children. These coefficients express the percentage variation of the child's blood pressure explained by the midparent blood pressure.

natural children and that of their natural parents, as shown on the left side of the figure. Indeed, the determination coefficient is 10.2 and 13.7% for the systolic and diastolic pressure, respectively ($p < 0.001$). In a very striking contrast, the correlation between adoptive midparent scores and that of the adopted children is very small and nonsignificant: 0.81% for the systolic and 1% for the diastolic.

Figure 3 shows the sib–sib correlation between natural children; the determination coefficient is 7.84% for systolic and 8.4% for diastolic blood pressure ($p < 0.05$). Again, the resemblance between pairs of adoptees is very small: 0.49% for systolic and 1.69% for diastolic.

Using a more sensitive statistical technique, the analysis of variance, the Fisher coefficient shows that the between-families variation of childhood pressure scores is significant at the 5% level for children of both statuses. However, the significance level of the difference is much higher for the natural children: $F = 2.96$ and 3.08 for systolic and diastolic blood pressure for the natural children ($p < 0.001$) and $F = 1.59$ and 1.52 for adopted children.

The correlation between randomly selected natural propositi and other siblings in families with more than one natural child was as follows: 4% for systolic and 9% for diastolic blood pressure. The same correlation among adopted children was much lower: 0.64% for systolic and 1.44% for diastolic blood pressure.

Because body weight seems to be a parameter often quoted as part of the etiology of hypertension, the correlation of body weight between parents and children was determined.

The midparent natural child correlation coefficient was 9.55% for body weight and 6.6% for weight/height ratio ($p = 0.0002$). The coefficients for midparents and adopted children were zero for body weight and zero for weight/height.

The natural sib–sib coefficients were 15.2% for body weight and 13.48% for

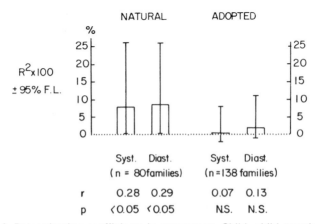

FIG. 3. Determination coefficients in percentage. Child–child correlations.

weight/height, and very highly significant ($p = 0.0003$), whereas the adopted child versus adopted child correlations were nonsignificant: 0.0047% for weight and 0.079% for weight/height.

Our data indicate that the blood pressure and the body size of a child resemble, to a small but significant degree, that of his natural parents, and that of his brothers and sisters. This is not the case for the adopted children.

Are these genetic characteristics affected by time? If we plot our correlation coefficients age by age, Fig. 4 shows that there is no increasing or decreasing trend as the child gets older. The correlation between natural children and their natural parents does not change with age. Therefore, our data suggest that the genetic influence of blood pressure and body size is stable before the age of 20.

Is the correlation between adopted children and adoptive parents influenced with time? Again, the age-by-age determination coefficient of our adopted

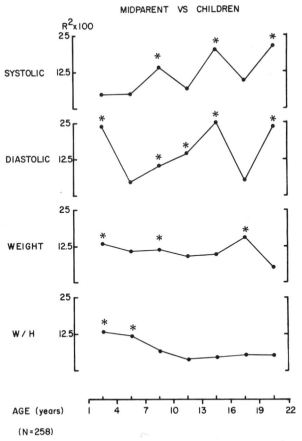

FIG. 4. Determination coefficients for natural children, plotted by age. The asterisks show that for this age group, the correlation is significantly greater than zero ($p < 0.05$).

children has no upward or downward trend observed along with the age. These results show that the environment did not significantly alter, with time, the resemblance of the adopted child's blood pressure and body size with that of his adoptive parents.

Finally, Dr. P. Philippe, a statistician of our institution, has estimated by more sophisticated statistical analysis that in the group of natural children, heredity was responsible for 94% and environment for 6% of the weight-resemblance findings. We are now working on a partial regression analysis whereby we will study the correlation of parent–child blood pressure, after taking into account the weight resemblance.

REFERENCES

1. DHEW Publication No. (HRA) 74-1617 (1973): Blood pressure levels of children 6–11 years. U.S. Department of Health, Education, and Welfare, Rockville, Md.
2. Moss, A. J., Adams, F. H. (1962): *Problems of Blood Pressure in Childhood*. Charles C Thomas, Springfield, Ill., pp. 66–83.

Juvenile Hypertension, edited by
M. I. New and L. S. Levine. Raven
Press, New York © 1977.

Does Hypertension Begin in Childhood? Studies of the Familial Aggregation of Blood Pressure in Childhood

*Stephen H. Zinner, **Harry S. Margolius, †Bernard R. Rosner, and †Edward H. Kass

*Department of Medicine, Roger Williams General Hospital, Brown University, Providence, Rhode Island 02908; **Departments of Pharmacology and Medicine, The Medical University of South Carolina, Charleston, South Carolina 29401; and †Channing Laboratory, Department of Medicine, Harvard Medical School, Boston City Hospital, Boston, Massachusetts 02118*

The etiology of essential hypertension remains unknown; however, it is reasonable to assume that factors responsible for the development of this disease are operative many years before the clinical onset of hypertensive signs and symptoms. As with any chronic disease, it is likely that the process of elevated blood pressure actually develops many decades before the signs and symptoms are manifest clinically. Also, it has been known for centuries that essential hypertension tends to cluster in families (1). More recently, detailed studies have suggested that family members of hypertensives have higher blood pressures than family members of nonhypertensives (2,3). The studies of Miall et al. (4) estimated the strength of the familial relation of blood pressures to be approximated by a regression coefficient of 0.3. Most of these studies involved adults, possibly because of the notion that blood pressures in children were unreliable or difficult to obtain.

In 1967, under the direction of Dr. Edward Kass at the Boston City Hospital, we began a systematic evaluation of blood pressures in children (5). This population was followed for a total of 8 years, and these studies form the basis of this report.

As these studies were in progress, a search was made for a biochemical factor that might correlate with blood pressure in these children. Because Margolius et al. (6) reported that urinary kallikrein excretion is decreased or absent in adults with untreated essential hypertension, urinary kallikrein was selected for epidemiological study in this population.

As a result of these and other studies, it may become possible to detect in childhood those families who are destined to develop essential hypertension when they reach their fourth and fifth decades.

MATERIALS AND METHODS

The initial population consisted of 721 children (aged 2 to 14 years) in 192 families in the Greater Boston area. These families were selected as part of a follow-up study of women who had been studied for bacteriuria in pregnancy in 1955 to 1959 (7–8). Approximately two-thirds of these women had been bacteriuric during their index pregnancy, and the remaining one-third were selected from a larger random sample of women who had not been bacteriuric at this time. Blood pressures were taken with the Kass-Mollo-Christensen blood pressure recorder (9). This device consists of a mercury sphygmomanometer, which is wired at 5-mm intervals to produce a square-wave signal on which the Korotkoff sounds are superimposed by a microphone placed in the antecubital fossa. When these signals are played through a single-channel recorder, a square-wave tracing is generated with the interval between each square wave representing 5 mm Hg (Fig. 1). The Korotkoff sounds appear as spikes; the pulses representing systolic and fourth- and fifth-phase diastolic pressures can be distinguished easily. This tracing forms a permanent record and can be read by several observers with an error between 2 and 3 mm Hg. All families were visited in their homes, and blood pressures were taken with this device after the children had been resting quietly for at least 5 min. In all studies, blood pressures were taken three times in succession, and the mean of the three readings was entered in the calculations.

All blood pressures were expressed as age- and sex-adjusted scores in standard deviation units (SDU) that are equal to the observed pressure for the individual minus the mean pressure for his 2-year age and sex group divided by the standard deviation of the blood pressures in this group.

In subsequent follow-up studies performed in 1970 to 1971 and in 1975, the

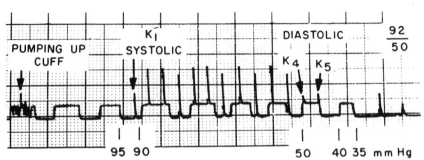

FIG. 1. Sample read-out tracing from automated blood pressure recorder. (From Kass and Zinner, ref. 9a.)

same procedure was used at the home visits and, in most cases, the same nurse involved in the original screening study measured the blood pressures of the children. At the second survey (1970 to 1971), a random urine specimen was obtained and stored at 4°C under toluene for the measurement of urinary kallikrein concentration. All kallikrein determinations were performed using a modification of the radioenzymatic method described by Beaven et al. (10). Statistical analysis employed included analysis of variance, single and multiple regression analysis and the chi-square test.

RESULTS—BLOOD PRESSURE STUDIES

When the blood pressure scores of the children at the initial visit were analyzed using the analysis of variance technique, it was found that the variance of blood pressure scores within families was significantly less than that among all children of this age group. This was reflected in an f score of 3.08 for systolic and 2.68 for diastolic pressures (Table 1). Thus, evidence of blood pressure clustering or the familial aggregation of blood pressure was demonstrated for children at least by age 2. Two subsequent studies at 3- to 4-year intervals revealed that the familial aggregation of blood pressure in these children remains essentially constant as they get older (Table 1).

In an attempt to determine the strength of this familial blood pressure relationship, sib–sib correlation coefficients were derived and reflected resemblance of blood pressures within these families. As seen in Table 2, the sib–sib correlation coefficient for systolic blood pressure was relatively similar for these children at each of three surveys.

In Fig. 2, mean family scores were calculated for each family by adjusting for family size; and when these scores were distributed, it was found that the distribution differed significantly from the normal distribution. This suggests that the familial aggregation of blood pressure operates over the entire range of blood pressures. It is of additional interest that approximately 8% of the families of children had blood pressure scores that were 2 SD or more above the mean. This finding led us to speculate as to the possibility that these

TABLE 1. *Familial aggregation of blood pressure in children at three surveys*

Survey	No. families	f scores[a]		
		Systolic[b]	$K_4{}^b$	K_5
1	192	3.08	2.68	—
2	163	1.97	2.02	1.83[b]
3	129	2.43	1.70	1.41[c]

[a]Blood pressure expressed in SDU.
[b]$p < 0.001$.
[c]$p < 0.01$.

TABLE 2. *Sib–sib correlation coefficients
for systolic blood pressure at three surveys*

Survey	No. children	r
1	721	0.34
2	609	0.21
3	485	0.28

children might become the hypertensives of the future. Follow-up studies of this population continued over an 8-year interval (11). As shown in Table 1, approximately 15% of families were lost to follow-up between each of these surveys. The familial aggregation of blood pressure did not differ for black versus white children and persisted when the blood pressure scores were adjusted for weight. Blood pressure itself was not significantly different for black and white children regardless of the age studied. This was true for all three surveys.

At the second survey, it was found that there was a significant positive relation of blood pressures obtained at this survey and those obtained initially (11). This was described by a regression coefficient of systolic blood pressure for the two surveys of 0.24, <0.001. As shown in Fig. 3, of the 88 children with initial scores greater than + 1 SDU, 57 or 65% had positive scores 4 years later. Preliminary data from the third survey suggest that the relation of previous blood pressures and the most recent pressures actually increases as

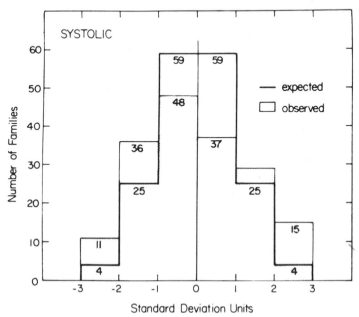

FIG. 2. Distribution of mean family scores for systolic blood pressure. (Reprinted by permission from *N. Engl. J. Med.*, 284:401–404, 1971, ref. 10a.)

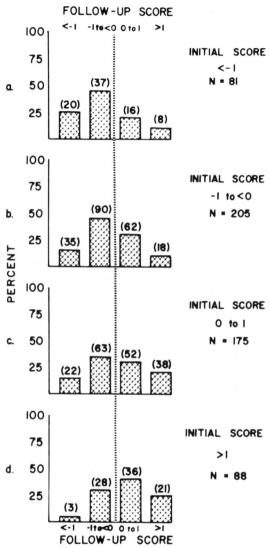

FIG. 3. Distribution of 4-year follow-up blood pressure scores in SDU according to initial score. Chi square, 40.447, *p* < 0.001. (From Zinner et al., ref. 11.)

the population ages. Thus, there is a tendency for stratification of blood pressure rank to begin in childhood and persist as the population ages, with higher pressures remaining relatively higher on subsequent surveys.

URINARY KALLIKREIN DETERMINATIONS

As seen in Table 3, the analysis of variance technique was applied to urinary kallikrein concentration (12) for 601 children in 163 families. The variance of

TABLE 3. *Analysis of variance—urinary kallikrein concentration*[a]

	DF	Mean square	f	p
Among families	162	1.851	3.45	< 0.001
Within families	438	0.536	—	—

[a]as logarithm.

these values within the families was significantly less than that among all children studied. Thus, urinary kallikrein concentration (expressed as the logarithm) appears to cluster in families at a strength similar to that observed for blood pressure. Of additional interest is the finding that urinary kallikrein concentration was significantly lower in black than in white children (logs: 3.922 versus 4.561, $p < 0.001$). This also was true when the data were adjusted for the other key variables that relate to urinary kallikrein.

The several additional variables found to relate significantly to urinary kallikrein concentration in these children included urinary potassium concentration ($b = 0.736$) and urinary creatinine concentration ($b = 0.335$). In general, urinary kallikrein concentration was higher when urine was obtained in the morning and was somewhat lower when obtained in the summer, as opposed to other times of the year. In addition, and of potential significance, is the finding that urinary kallikrein concentration was inversely related to diastolic blood pressure both in the children and in the mother. Ten percent of the families with the lowest mean kallikrein concentration had significantly higher blood pressure scores than did the 10% of families with the highest kallikrein concentrations (12).

DISCUSSION

The results of these studies suggest several possible conclusions. First, it is clear that blood pressure per se can be shown to aggregate in families of children as early as 2 years of age. This strong familial clustering effect is reproducible when these children are studied over an 8-year period. In addition, it has been demonstrated that there is a significant and positive relation of blood pressures in these children as the population ages and is restudied. In fact, the increasing regression coefficients for subsequent surveys imply that there might be some environmental influences responsible for the closer relation of successive blood pressure readings in time.

The relation of rising blood pressures with age remains controversial. Miall and Lovell (13) presented data suggesting that the rate of rise of pressure depends on "attained" pressure with a steeper, more rapid rise for those pressures already elevated above the mean. Other studies have suggested that adults with "high normal" pressures continue to exhibit, with time, a tendency toward higher pressures (14,15). Whether or not the children in our studies, whose blood pressures are 2 SD or more above the mean for their age, will in fact develop hypertension when they reach middle age cannot be determined now. However, additional measurements of this population do show the tendency for higher pressures to persist after a 7- to 8-year study period.

An understanding of the natural history of blood pressures in children is just beginning. Virtually no data exist with respect to the predictive value of neonatal blood pressures on pressures later in life. Lee et al. (16) and Klein et al. (17) suggested that familial blood pressure relations can be demonstrated at birth or in the early months of life. It is now possible from the data presented to begin to hypothesize that blood pressure "tracking" may begin in childhood. It is also conceivable that this tracking phenomenon may extend into the newborn. "Tracking" describes the assumption that once one's blood pressure has entered a track (e.g., high for age or low for age), it tends to continue along that track with time so that higher pressures remain higher. Since there is not usually a crisis onset of high blood pressure in adults, it is reasonable to assume that children with relatively high blood pressures for their age (even though still within the normal range) are more likely to develop essential hypertension when they reach middle age.

Currently, it is not possible to predict with accuracy, given an individual child or family of children, that in fact these children are at greater risk of essential hypertension when they reach adulthood. However, it is possible that low urinary kallikrein concentration or excretion might be a useful marker to detect high-risk children. The data presented suggest strongly that urinary kallikrein concentration is considerably lower in black than in white children. We have not been able to demonstrate that blood pressures in these children are higher in black than in white children. However, it is well known that black adults generally have higher blood pressures and a greater frequency of clinical hypertension than white adults (18–20). It is possible that the racial difference in urinary kallikrein might precede the racial difference in blood pressure. Whether the kallikrein–kinin system is related to the subsequent development of hypertension or, in fact, to the regulation of blood pressure itself cannot be stated at this time. However, further studies need to be directed in this area to determine if, in fact, the associations presented have any bearing on the subsequent development of high blood pressure.

The factors responsible for the elevation of blood pressure have not been identified. However, it appears logical that these should be sought as close as possible to the time of onset of elevated pressures. Large-scale studies of the familial aggregation of blood pressures directed at infants and children are likely to shed light in this area and should be of interest in evaluating etiologic factors in the pathogenesis of essential hypertension. Finally, it is entirely possible that essential hypertension begins and is potentially detectable in childhood or earlier. The possibility of potential intervention in childhood to prevent the inexorable rise of pressure over many decades remains an exciting challenge for future research.

ACKNOWLEDGMENTS

This work was supplemented by a grant-in-aid from the American Heart Association with funds contributed in part by the Greater Boston Heart Association, and by Research Grant HDO3693 from the National Institute of Child Health and Human Development.

REFERENCES

1. Morgagni, J. B. (1761): *De sedibus, et causus morborum per anatomen indagatis,* Vol. 1. Remondiniana, Venice.
2. Ayman, D. (1934): Heredity in arteriolar (essential) hypertension: A clinical study of the blood pressure of 1,524 members of 277 families. *Arch. Intern. Med.,* 53:792–802.
3. Gearing, F. R., Clark, E. G., Perera, G. A., and Schweitzer, M. D. (1962): Hypertension among relatives of hypertensives: Progress report of a family study. *Am. J. Public Health,* 52:2058–2065.
4. Miall, W. E., Heneage, P., Khosla, T., Lovell, H. G., and Moore, F. (1967): Factors influencing the degree of resemblance in arterial pressure of close relatives. *Clin. Sci. Mol. Med.,* 33:271–283.
5. Zinner, S. H., Levy, P. S., and Kass, E. H. (1971): Familial aggregation of blood pressure in childhood. *N. Engl. J. Med.,* 284:401–404.
6. Margolius, H. S., Geller, R., Pisano, J. J., and Sjoerdsma, A. (1971): Altered urinary kallikrein excretion in human hypertension. *Lancet,* 2:1063–1065.
7. Zinner, S. H., and Kass, E. H. (1971): Longterm (10–15 years) followup of bacteriuria of pregnancy. *N. Engl. J. Med.,* 285:820–824.
8. Savage, W. E., Hajj, S. N., and Kass, E. H. (1967): Demographic and prognostic characteristics of bacteriuria in pregnancy. *Medicine (Balt.),* 46:385–407.
9. Zinner, S. H., Taylor, J. O., Rosner, B., Mark, R., Zimmerman, D., and Kass, E. H. (1972): Comparison of an automated blood pressure recorder with a random zero sphygmomanometer. *Clin. Res.,* 20:206.
9a. Kass, E. H., and Zinner, S. H. (1969): How early can the tendency for hypertension be detected. *Milbank Mem. Fund Q.,* 47(2):143–152.
10. Beaven, V. H., Pierce, J. V., and Pisano, J. J. (1971): A sensitive isotopic procedure for the assay of esterase activity: Measurement of urinary kallikrein. *Clin. Chim. Acta* 32:67–73.
10a. Zinner, S. H., Levy, P. S., and Kass, E. H. (1971): Familial aggregation of blood pressure in childhood. *N. Engl. J. Med.,* 284:401–404.
11. Zinner, S. H., Martin, L. F., Sacks, F., Rosner, B. and Kass, E. H. (1975): A longitudinal study of blood pressure in childhood. *Am. J. Epidemiol.,* 100:437–442.
12. Zinner, S. H., Margolius, H. S., Rosner, B., Keiser, H. R., and Kass, E. H. (1976): Familial aggregation of urinary kallikrein concentration in childhood; relation to blood pressure, race and urinary electrolytes. *Am. J. Epidemiol.,* 104:124–132.
13. Miall, W. E., and Lovell, H. G. (1967): Relation between change of blood pressure and age. *Br. Med. J.,* 2:660–664.
14. Feinleib, M., Gordon, T., Garrison, R. J., Kannel, W. B., and Verter, J. I. (1969): Blood pressure and age: The Framingham Study. In: *Second Annual Meeting of the Society for Epidemiological Research, Chapel Hill, N.C., May 3.*
15. Harlan, W. R., Oberman, A., Mitchell, R. W., and Graybiel, A. (1971): A thirty year study of blood pressure in a white male cohort. *Clin. Res.,* 19:319.
16. Lee, Y. H., Rosner, B., Gould, J. B., and Kass, E. H. (1976): Familial aggregation of blood pressures of newborn infants and their mothers. *Pediatrics, in press.*
17. Klein, B. E., Hennekens, C. H., Jesse, M. J., Gourley, J. E., and Blumenthal, S. (1975): Longitudinal studies of blood pressure in offspring of hypertensive mothers. In: *Epidemiology and Control of Hypertension,* edited by O. Paul. Stratton Corp., New York.
18. McDonough, J. R., Garrison, G. E., and Hames, C. G. (1964): Blood pressure and hyperten-

sive disease among Negroes and whites; a study in Evans County, Georgia. *Ann. Intern. Med.,* 61:208–228.

19. Comstock, G. W. (1957): An epidemiologic study of blood pressure levels in a biracial community in the southern United States. *Am. J. Hygiene,* 65:271–315.
20. Johnson, B. C., and Remington, R. D. (1961): A sampling study of blood pressure levels in white and Negro residents of Nassau, Bahamas. *J. Chronic Dis.,* 13:39–51.

Juvenile Hypertension, edited by
M. I. New and L. S. Levine. Raven
Press, New York © 1977.

Comment: Hereditary Nature of Blood Pressure and Hypertension in Children

Lenore S. Levine

A number of studies have documented the importance of family history in the development of essential hypertension in childhood[1-4] or in later life [5,6]. The studies presented in this section demonstrate the highly significant influence of genetics, not only in hypertension but also in determining blood pressure per se; they also demonstrate that the genetic effect is present even in early childhood and is more significant than environmental factors.

The relationship between kallikrein excretion and blood pressure requires continued evaluation.

[1]Levine, L. S., Lewy, J. E., and New, M. I. (1976): Hypertension in high school students; evaluation in New York City. *N.Y. State J. Med.,* 76(1):40–44.

[2]Haggerty, R. J., Maroney, M. W., and Nadas, A. S. (1956): Essential hypertension in infancy and childhood, differential diagnosis and therapy. *Am. J. Dis. Child.,* 92:535–549.

[3]Singh, S. P., and Page, L. B. (1967): Hypertension in early life. *Am. J. Med. Sci.,* 253:255–262.

[4]Londe, S., Bourgoignie, J. J., Robson, A. M., and Goldring, D. (1971): Hypertension in apparently normal children. *J. Pediatr.,* 78:569–577.

[5]Paffenbarger, R. S., Jr., Thorne, M. C., and Wing, S. L. (1968): Chronic disease in former college students. VIII. Characteristics in youth predisposing to hypertension in later years. *Am. J. Epidemiol.,* 88:25–32.

[6]Friman, G., and Waern, U. (1974): Blood pressure and blood lipids in members of families with a heavy aggregation of essential hypertension. *Acta Med. Scand.,* 196:11–16.

Juvenile Hypertension, edited by
M. I. New and L. S. Levine. Raven
Press, New York © 1977.

Adrenocortical Secretory Activity in Genetic and Experimental Hypertension

James C. Melby, Anthony L. McCall, and Sidney L. Dale

Section of Endocrinology and Metabolism, Department of Medicine, Boston University School of Medicine, University Hospital, Boston, Massachusetts 02118

There exist several animal models in which hypertension is associated with adrenal secretory abnormalities, alterations in adrenocortical morphology, and dependence on anterior pituitary function. The models to be described in this report were observed in rats in whom hypertension was induced experimentally or occurred spontaneously, because of genetic predisposition. Three models will be described: adrenal regeneration hypertension, androgen-induced hypertension, and spontaneous hypertension of genetic origin. In all three of these models, alterations in steroid biosynthesis were observed and seem to be intimately related to the appearance of hypertension. In these models, excessive salt ingestion speeds the onset of hypertension and intensifies the hypertensive diathesis. The combination of excessive mineralocorticoid activity and the presence of increased salt ingestion lead to expansion of the extracellular fluid volume and, ultimately, to hypertension. The mineralocorticoid–hypertensive syndrome, which can be shown to exist in adrenal regeneration hypertension and in rats treated with androgen, is invariably associated with inhibition of the renin–angiotensin system because of increased sodium content of biological fluids and expansion of the extracellular fluid volume. In this chapter, rat models of experimental and genetic hypertension will be described and evidence presented, either conclusive or incomplete, that mineralocorticoid hyperactivity plays some role in the development of the hypertensive state.

ADRENAL REGENERATION HYPERTENSION

The development of severe hypertensive disease that occurs in the rat following unilateral adrenalectomy and nephrectomy, and contralateral adrenal enucleation, was first described by Skelton (1). The mechanism by which

57

the regenerating adrenal initiates the hypertension is not known; however, it is likely that secretion of one or more adrenocortical steroids is essential to the initiation and perpetuation of the hypertension. Hypophysectomy (2) and suppression of endogenous corticotropin secretion by exogenous corticosterone administration (3) block the development of hypertension. Thus, it would appear that steroidogenesis by the regenerating adrenal is ACTH dependent. Mineralocorticoid antagonists also prevent the hypertension sequence (4).

The offending steroid is not aldosterone, because secretion is markedly diminished during the development of hypertension. Rapp (4) found peripheral blood deoxycorticosterone (DOC) levels elevated after the establishment of hypertension and failed to find elevations of peripheral blood 18-hydroxy-11-deoxycorticosterone (18-OH-DOC) concentrations. Birmingham et al. (5) observed that regenerating adrenal slices incubated *in vitro* elaborated more 18-OH-DOC with ACTH stimulation than did slices of adrenal glands from normal rats. Because of these seemingly conflicting observations, adrenal regeneration hypertension was studied by sampling adrenal venous effluent at various intervals after the enucleation procedure.

In a series of studies reported from this laboratory (6,7), it was demonstrated that the secretion of all steroids into the adrenal venous effluent of rats with adrenal regeneration hypertension was markedly decreased within 24 hr of the enucleation. DOC secretion began to rise at 1 week and returned to near control levels at 3 weeks after enucleation. 18-OH-DOC secretion was markedly diminished during the first 3 weeks but greatly oversecreted in the 3 weeks after enucleation. Corticosterone secretion returned to normal at 6 weeks and aldosterone secretion remained low throughout the study, but it must be recalled that these animals are ingesting larger amounts of sodium chloride. These studies on direct adrenal secretion of steroids suggest that conflicting previous studies may nearly reflect sampling or experimental procedures carried out at differing times during the time-course development of adrenal regeneration hypertension. In Fig. 1, secretion of 18-OH-DOC and DOC by enucleated adrenals is compared over 6 weeks, and it is clearly seen that 18-OH-DOC excess is present at 6 weeks and that restoration of DOC secretion is obvious by 3 weeks.

Peripheral steroid levels, obtained in the basal or unstressed state in rats during the development of adrenal regeneration hypertension, confirmed the suspicions aroused by the adrenal venous effluent data that both DOC and 18-OH-DOC were involved in the production of adrenal regeneration hypertension. Gaunt et al. (8) have clearly demonstrated that basal peripheral DOC levels are at least 10-fold greater in the enucleate animals, as compared with controls, at 3 weeks following enucleation. It is at this time that the animals are frankly hypertensive. It should be pointed out that DOC levels begin to increase in the peripheral blood at approximately 2 weeks. In Fig. 2, peripheral levels of 18-OH-DOC and DOC are represented diagrammatically during the development of adrenal regeneration hypertension. It can be seen that 18-

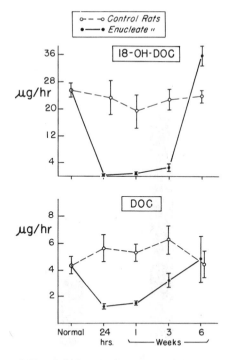

FIG. 1. Steroid secretion in control and enucleate rats during the development of adrenal regeneration hypertension.

OH-DOC levels in the peripheral blood are greatly increased at 6 weeks; whereas DOC levels, as previously stated, are greatly increased at 3 weeks. Since significant hypertension is clearly evident by 3 weeks in these animals, at a time when peripheral DOC concentrations are markedly elevated, it is highly likely that DOC is the inciting steroid for the onset of hypertension. It is equally likely that excessive secretion of 18-OH-DOC perpetuates and worsens adrenal regeneration hypertension at a time when all other mineralocorticoid secretion is, if anything, suppressed. It should be emphasized that the amount of 18-OH-DOC, which is secreted in the enucleate rat with adrenal regeneration hypertension, exceeds by far the amount necessary to produce hypertension by injection of exogenous 18-OH-DOC.

ANDROGEN-INDUCED HYPERTENSION

Floyd Skelton first demonstrated that methylandrostenediol injections in the rat could produce severe hypertension, especially when the rats were sensitized by previous uninephrectomy and increased salt ingestion. Brownie and Skelton (9) were able to demonstrate that methylandrostenediol induced inhibition of 11β- and 18-hydroxylations and that the result was an overproduction of DOC or 18-OH-DOC, with consequent reduction in secretion of corticosterone. Evidence for the inhibition of the 18-hydroxylation pathway was adduced from radiolabeled precursor product studies. Colby et al. (10)

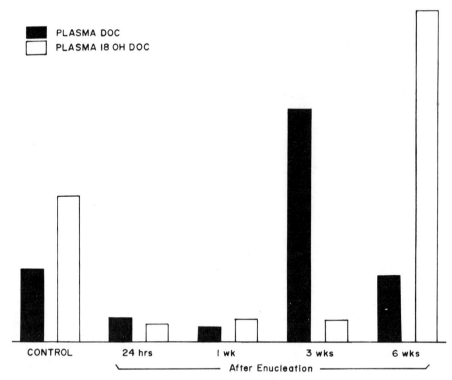

FIG. 2. Peripheral levels of plasma DOC and plasma 18-OH-DOC during the development of adrenal regeneration hypertension. Results are expressed diagrammatically.

were able to induce hypertension in uninephrectomized female rats given 10 mg of testosterone, daily, for 35 days; the rats also received additional salt. It was demonstrated that testosterone treatment resulted in increased conversion of labeled precursors by adrenal tissues *in vitro* to DOC and diminished conversion to corticosterone and 18-OH-DOC. Testosterone-induced hypertension in the rat seems to be mediated by the same mechanism as that of methylandrostenediol. DOC excess would appear to be the inciting cause of hypertension in each instance. It may be surmised that cessation of testosterone administration would not alter the development of the hypertensive diathesis, because of the occurrence of so-called metacorticoid hypertension.

Metacorticoid hypertension refers to the irreversible progress of hypertension after mineralocorticoid administration. For example, DOC may be given for a period of 4 to 6 weeks to susceptible rats, and after the cessation of DOC administration, these animals remain hypertensive. In fact, the hypertension worsens and severe vascular complications ensue. The mechanism of metacorticoid hypertension has not been elucidated but it is of great current interest, because it is possible that brief hypersecretion of mineralocorticoids could induce a permanent hypertensive state. This appears to be the case in patients who remain hypertensive after the removal of an aldosterone-producing adenoma.

The existence of metacorticoid hypertension emphasizes the need for studies on the time course of hormonal steroid secretory activity during the genesis of the hypertensive state. Any study purporting to exclude mineralocorticoid excess as a determinant of the hypertensive state must provide evidence of unaltered steroid secretory activity during the entire period of genesis of hypertension. The obvious possibility arises that transient increments in DOC secretion could occur in human subjects during periods of excessive androgen production (puberty, etc.), with the development of hypertension. Time course of androgen-altered secretion of adrenal steroidogenesis was studied in this laboratory, in detail, and is the subject of a report to be published elsewhere by McCall et al. (11). The principal findings of these studies include the characterization of adrenal steroidogenesis *in vivo* by sequential adrenal vein catheterizations during the development of methylandrostenediol-induced hypertension. In this study, uninephrectomy was not carried out but 1% saline was given as drinking solution. Androgen-treated rats were hypertensive by 6 weeks of 10-mg injections, daily, of methylandrostenediol. Adrenal secretion of corticosterone, DOC, 18-OH-DOC, and aldosterone was measured by catheterizing adrenal veins at 2, 4, 6, and 8 weeks.

In Fig. 3, it can be seen that DOC secretion, as expected, rose sharply; at 2 weeks it exceeded the control by severalfold and at 4 weeks declined thereafter, approaching control levels by the 8th week. 18-OH-DOC levels fell during treatment but approached control levels by the 8th week. Corticosterone secretion was markedly depressed in the androgen-treated group as compared to the controls. Aldosterone secretion, although depressed at 2 and 4 weeks, approached control levels at 6 and 8 weeks. It appears that androgen produces a profound alteration in adrenal steroidogenesis and that the abnormal excessive production of DOC precedes the onset of hypertension and wanes while the animals remain hypertensive.

It is likely that, in these studies, the androgen-treated rat has entered the metacorticoid phase of hypertension. It is not known whether androgens in high doses stimulate DOC secretion in man. These investigations were undertaken at this laboratory in the last year. It is unlikely that mature males would exhibit much effect to excessive androgen administration because of their prior endogenous exposure. It is possible that pubertal males may exhibit transient increments in DOC levels and this needs to be examined.

SPONTANEOUSLY HYPERTENSIVE RATS

Despite much research on the pathogenesis of hypertension in spontaneously hypertensive rats (SHR) in the past, the etiology remains obscure. Morphological evidence of hyperactivity of the pituitary–adrenal axis was demonstrated in the pathological studies of Aoki et al. (12). More recently,

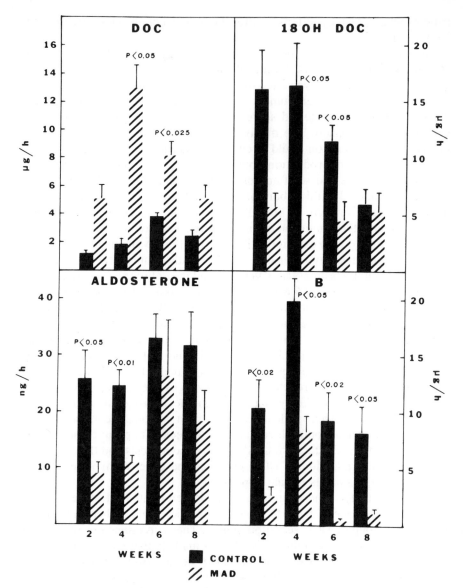

FIG. 3. Steroid secretion in control and methylandrostenediol (MAD)-treated rats during the development of hypertension.

Tabei et al. (13) have shown that, on electron microscopy, the zona fasciculata of the SHR adrenal resembles that seen with chronic ACTH stimulation, and there is morphological evidence of increased secretory activity of ACTH producing pituitary cells. Other studies have suggested the involvement of a mineralocorticoid. These include low juxtaglomerular indices in the kidneys of

SHR (14), low renal renin in the advanced hypertensive stage (15), as well as low plasma potassium, as compared to controls.

Adrenal ablation studies have raised controversy over the role of the adrenal. Aoki (16) showed that bilateral adrenalectomy could prevent the development of hypertension in the prehypertensive stage and reduce blood pressure to normal in the hypertensive stage in animals given saline to drink. In contrast to these studies, Baer et al. (17) showed that in the early hypertensive SHR, bilateral adrenalectomy did not prevent further increase in blood pressure, although it rose more slowly than controls.

In our laboratory, Moll et al. (18), to further elucidate the role of the adrenal in hypertension of SHR, studied steroidogenesis sequentially by means of adrenal vein catheterization at different ages during the development of hypertension.

Figure 4 shows the body weight, blood pressure, and adrenal weight of the rats used. Body weights were less in SHR than in age-matched controls. Blood pressures of SHR are higher than controls, even in young animals, and begin to rise to hypertensive levels by 13 weeks of age. By 20 weeks of age, SHR blood pressures are in the range of 170 mm Hg, while controls have remained at the 115- to 120-mm level. Adrenal weights are not significantly different in the two groups.

Figures 5 and 6 represent, by means of bar graphs, the adrenal secretion rate data for DOC and 18-OH-DOC of SHR at different ages as compared to controls during the development of hypertension. The secretion of aldosterone is significantly lower in SHR at 8 weeks of age. As the animals grew older, we could demonstrate no significant difference in the secretion rate of aldosterone at ages 12, 15, and 20 weeks.

The secretion rate of DOC is not different in young SHR as compared to controls up to 15 weeks of age. At 20 weeks of age, DOC secretion is significantly depressed. The secretion of 18-OH-DOC was reduced in young SHR, a significant difference being demonstrated at 12 weeks. As the SHR became older, they seemed to be producing greater amounts of 18-OH-DOC. In the 20-week-old animals, no significant difference in 18-OH-DOC secretion could be demonstrated between SHR and controls.

Corticosterone secretion showed no significant difference at 8 weeks, when the animals were not hypertensive. As the animals developed hypertension, we found corticosterone secretion significantly reduced at ages 12 and 20 weeks. Secretion data suggest either an enzyme block or an increased conversion of known steroids to an unknown steroid product. Reduced secretion of corticosterone could explain the adrenal hyperplasia observed in SHR, which may be important to the development of hypertension in these animals.

Adrenal regeneration hypertension and androgen-induced hypertension in the rat appear to be initiated by oversecretion of DOC. Hypersecretion of DOC in androgen-induced hypertension is a transitory phenomenon, yet sufficient in duration to produce permanent progressive hypertension. In

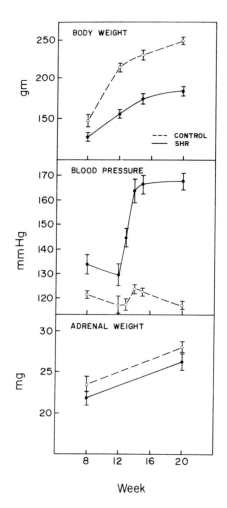

FIG. 4. Body weights, blood pressures, and adrenal weights of SHR and control rats at different ages. Vertical bars indicate + or − SE (*n* = six rats).

adrenal regeneration hypertension, hypersecretion of DOC is extremely brief and is supplanted by excessive secretion of 18-OH-DOC, which probably serves to intensify and perpetuate the hypertensive diathesis and assure the development of metacorticoid hypertension. Brief transitory exposure to hypersecretion of mineralocorticoids cannot be dismissed as a possible predisposing factor in the development of hypertension in the young. Studies in pubertal human males are needed to determine whether physiological hypersecretion of androgen induces transitory DOC secretory excess.

Alterations in steroid biogenesis in SHR are clearly seen at 20 weeks, when nearly all of the colony is hypertensive. In these animals, evidence of ACTH oversecretion, adrenal enlargement, and depressed secretion of corticosterone, 18-OH-DOC, and other steroids suggest that there is, perhaps, some

DEOXYCORTICOSTERONE (DOC)

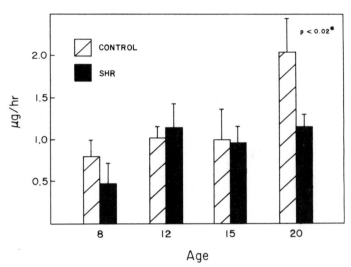

FIG. 5. Adrenal secretion of DOC in SHR and control rats. Data are expressed as per adrenal gland.

18 - OH - DOC

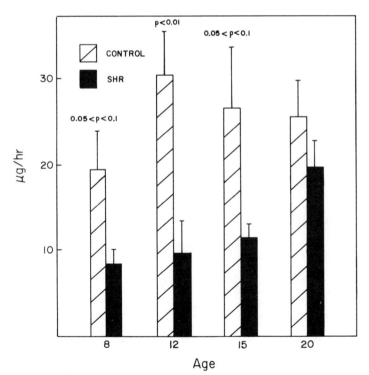

FIG. 6. Adrenal secretion rates of 18-OH-DOC in SHR and control rats. Data are expressed as per adrenal gland.

abnormal steroid being produced. Evidence for an unusual or, heretofore, undescribed steroid is lacking. It is tempting to speculate that the 11β- and 18-hydroxylations are somehow disturbed in this condition and that there exists oversecretion of 11-deoxysteroids, such as DOC, sometimes initiating the onset of hypertension. For these studies, it will be necessary to examine the peripheral plasma concentrations of DOC in the quiescent SHR. The role of the adrenal cortex in the genesis of some forms of experimental and genetic hypertension in the rat appears to be established.

ACKNOWLEDGMENTS

This work was supported by Grants-in-Aid #AM 12027-09, PO2-AM-08657-12, and HL-18318-01 (SRC) from the National Institutes of Health.

REFERENCES

1. Skelton, F. R. (1955): Development of hypertension and cardiovascular-renal lesions during adrenal regeneration in the rat. *Proc. Soc. Exp. Biol. Med.,* 90:342–346.
2. Skelton, F. R. (1956): Adrenal regeneration hypertension and factors influencing its development. *Arch. Intern. Med.,* 98:449–462.
3. Skelton, F. R. (1958): Production and inhibition of hypertensive disease in the rat by corticosterone. *Endocrinology,* 62:365–368.
4. Rapp, J. P. (1969): Deoxycorticosterone production in adrenal regeneration hypertension: *In vitro* vs *in vivo* comparison. *Endocrinology,* 84:1409–1420.
5. Birmingham, M. K., MacDonald, M. L., and Rochefort, J. G. (1968): Adrenal function in normal rats and in rats bearing regenerated adrenal glands. In: *Functions of the Adrenal Cortex,* Vol. II, edited by K. W. McKerns, pp. 647–689. Appleton-Century-Crofts, New York.
6. Melby, J. C., Dale, S. L., Grekin, R. J., Gaunt, R., and Wilson, T. E. (1972): 18-Hydroxy-11-deoxycorticosterone (18-OH-DOC) secretion in experimental and human hypertension. *Recent Prog. Horm. Res.,* 28:287–351.
7. Grekin, R. J., Dale, S. L., Gaunt, R., and Melby, J. C. (1972): Steroid secretion by the enucleated rat adrenal: Measurements during salt retention and the development of hypertension. *Endocrinology,* 91(5):1166–1171.
8. Gaunt, R., Melby, J. C., Dale, S. L., Grekin, R., and Brown, R. (1972): Adrenal regeneration hypertension. In: *Proc. 4th Intn'l Congr. Endocrinology, Amsterdam, The Netherlands,* pp. 18–24. Excerpta Medica, Amsterdam.
9. Brownie, A. C., and Skelton, F. R. (1968): Adrenocortical Function and Structure in Adrenal Regeneration Hypertension and Methylandrostenediol Hypertension. In: *Functions of the Adrenal Cortex,* Vol. II, edited by K. W. McKerns, pp. 691–718. Appleton-Century-Crofts, New York.
10. Colby, H. D., Skelton, F. R., and Brownie, A. C. (1970): Testosterone-induced hypertension in the rat. *Endocrinology,* 86:1093–1101.
11. McCall, A., Dale, S. L., and Melby, J. C. (1976): Adrenal steroidogenesis in androgen-induced hypertension. *Endocrinology, submitted for publication.*
12. Aoki, K. H., Tankawa, T., Fujinami, A., Miyazaki, A., and Hashimoto, Y. (1963): Pathological studies on the endocrine organs of the spontaneously hypertensive rats. *Jpn. Heart J.,* 4:426–442.
13. Tabei, R., Maruyama, T., Kumada, M., and Okamoto, K. (1972): Morphological studies on endocrine organs in spontaneously hypertensive rats. In: *Spontaneous Hypertention,* edited by K. Okamoto, p. 185–193. Igaku Shoin Ltd., Tokyo.

14. Koletsky, S., Shook, P., and Rivera-Valez, J. (1972): Absence of hyperactive renal humoral pressor system in spontaneously hypertensive rats. In: *Spontaneous Hypertention,* edited by K. Okamoto, p. 199–202. Igaku Shoin Ltd., Tokyo.
15. Sokabe, H. (1966): Renin activity of the kidney in the spontaneously hypertensive rat. *Jpn. J. Physiol.,* 16:380–388.
16. Aoki, K. (1963): Experimental studies on the relationship between endocrine organs and hypertension in spontaneously hypertensive rats. *Jpn. Heart J.,* 4:443–461.
17. Baer, L., Knowton, A., and Laragh, J. H. (1972): The role of sodium balance and the pituitary-adrenal axis in the hypertension of spontaneously hypertensive rats. In: *Spontaneous Hypertension,* edited by K. Okamoto, p. 203–209. Igaku Shoin Ltd., Tokyo.
18. Moll, D., Dale, S. L., and Melby, J. C. (1975): Adrenal steroidogenesis in the spontaneously hypertensive rat. *Endocrinology,* 96(2):416–420.

Juvenile Hypertension, edited by
M. I. New and L. S. Levine. Raven
Press, New York © 1977.

Further Studies on the ACTH-Induced Hypertension in Sheep: Involvement of New Hypertensinogenic Steroid Hormones

J. P. Coghlan, D. A. Denton, J. S. K. Fan, J. G. McDougall, and B. A. Scoggins

Howard Florey Institute of Experimental Physiology and Medicine, University of Melbourne, Parkville 3052, Australia

In light of the long-standing interest of our scientific group in sodium metabolism, and its central place in any discussion of hypertension, we had felt that it would be appropriate here to consider the issue of chronic and sustained excess salt intake in the possible etiology of hypertension. In other words, we will elaborate on the arguments for and against the proposal that the appetite and conservation mechanisms of sodium homeostasis that have emerged over the 30 million years of primate evolution have done so under generally prevailing conditions of sodium scarcity (6). For the majority of homo sapiens, salt has become relatively cheap and abundant only as a result of the technology and commerce of the last 100 years.

The phylogenetic legacy is one of scarcity. Hedonic or pleasure elements of appetite (7) have conferred considerable survival advantage during tropical existence and conditions of scarcity. However, these same elements may now determine sustained excess intake unrelated to metabolic need, over the course of life. This could be important in genetically susceptible individuals, with or without other contributory hypertensinogenic factors, on a chronic basis. In this context, attention must be given to the studies carried out in primitive communities—most recently the Tukisenta of highland New Guinea (23) and the Yanamamo Indians of Venezuela and Brazil (16)—where no blood pressure rise occurs in the population with the aging process. An outstanding feature of the life style in both instances, as with other similar communities, is the very low-sodium intake and high potassium/sodium ratio in the predominantly vegetarian diet.

There is evidence to support the proposal that chronic high-salt intake, quite unrelated to dietetic need, is one of the examples in a growing dossier of damage caused by subtle long-term effects of excess of substances that are normal, indeed essential, components of diet. If this is so, then much emphasis should be placed on the fact that these effects may be most damaging in infancy and childhood, a period in which habituation and conditioning to high-salt taste patterns may develop and then persist for life. The influence on the structure and response characteristics of tissues may be maximal during the period of most rapid growth. Dahl's studies on young rats (5) suggest that this may be true, specifically in relation to salt and blood pressure.

Bearing the above evidence in mind, but also the fact that essential hypertension in western man is a complex problem with a jointly sufficient and severally necessary causal basis rather than any simple effect, we feel it appropriate to center this chapter on the question of a new hypertensinogenic steroid of the adrenal gland. It will open up some interesting new avenues of experimental analysis of hypertension, and may conceivably throw some light on human hypertension in both adults and children (14). In our experimental analysis to be presented, the influence of sodium status on the process will be a major issue.

Our model of hypertension, one of rapid onset and reversibility, involves the administration of exogenous ACTH. ACTH administration of 80 IU/day to intact conscious sheep causes a significant elevation of arterial blood pressure within 24 hr, and this is sustained as long as ACTH is given over a 5- to 10-day period (Fig. 1, Group E). Hypokalemia, an increase in plasma sodium, and an

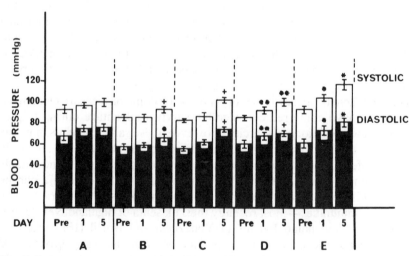

FIG. 1. Group **A:** mean systolic and diastolic blood pressure (± SEM) before (pre) and after 1 and 5 days of the combined steroid infusion. Group **B:** combined steroid plus 18-OH-DOC. Group **C:** combined steroid plus 17 α-OHP. Group **D:** combined steroid plus 17α,20α-diOHP. Group **E:** combined steroid plus ACTH. Statistical comparisons with control (pre) observations were made using the Student's *t*-test for paired observations. *, $p < 0.05$; **, $p < 0.01$; +, $p < 0.005$.

increased water intake and urine output were also observed. The sustained increases in blood pressure were not, however, related to changes in the external sodium status, body weight, or the renin–angiotensin system. This ACTH-induced increase in blood pressure is dependent on the presence of adrenal glands but not on intact adrenal innervation (22). It is associated with an increase in cardiac output and rate and an increase in plasma volume, although not in extracellular fluid space (20).

Intravenous infusion of cortisol, 11-deoxycortisol, corticosterone, deoxy-corticosterone (DOC), and aldosterone, either singly or in combination at rates to give blood levels similar to those measured during ACTH administration (Fig. 1, Group A), failed to reproduce the elevation in blood pressure. This combined steroid infusion did reproduce all the other metabolic responses found to be characteristic of ACTH treatment (8, 19). In other experiments where the combined steroid infusion was given, but with a high level of aldosterone (10 to 20 μg/hr) over the first 24 hr, there was no increase in blood pressure. Furthermore, spironolactone (Aldactone®, G. D. Searle), a drug used clinically as a mineralocorticoid antagonist, when given intravenously at 400 mg/day for 5 days to animals undergoing ACTH treatment, reversed the electrolyte changes but did not lower blood pressure.

The fact that the adrenal cortex may be involved in the pathogenesis of hypertension originated from the autopsy observation on two patients by Neussen in 1897 (13); this was supported in 1924 by Oppenheimer and Fishberg (18) in a larger series. Thereafter, hypertension associated with excessive endogenous steroid production or administration of exogenous steroids has been widely reported in both clinical and experimental studies. Although the cause(s) of increased blood pressure in some of these studies is well known, in others it is not yet clear. Historically, two classes of steroids—mineralocorticoids (e.g., aldosterone, DOC, and corticosterone) and gluco-corticoids (e.g., cortisol and 11-deoxycortisol)—have been thought to cause hypertension. The exact mechanism by which these types of hypertension are produced and the precise relationship between these steroids, sodium status, and blood pressure are still largely undefined. In addition, since the birth of "low renin essential hypertension" in the early 1960s (2,10), volume expansion as a result of increased secretion of an unidentified mineralocorticoid has been raised as a possibility by several groups (1,3,4,9,11,24,26,27); it is against this background that Melby and co-workers (12) set out in search of new hypertensinogenic steroids. To date, naturally occurring steroids, for example, 18-hydroxydeoxycorticosterone (18-OH-DOC), 16,18-dihydroxydeoxy-corticosterone (16,18-diOH-DOC), and 16β-hydroxydehydroepiandrosterone (16β-OH-DHEA), have been investigated for their hypertensive activities (12,21). The first has been found to increase blood pressure in the dog (17) and sheep (8), whereas any hypertensinogenic action of the latter requires confirmation. In our model of hypertension, allowing that the hypertension is dependent on adrenal secretion, it is logical to explore the possibilities of the different steroids during the development of hypertension, including those actually measured as increased in adrenal vein blood. Therefore, several steroids have been infused with the combined steroid infusion that, as noted above, by itself was not hypertensive. Preliminary experiments with 16β-OH-DHEA at 200 μg/hr with the combined steroid solution had no effect on blood pressure. The combined steroid infusion together with 18-OH-DOC at 100 μg/hr, which is probably a pharmacological level in the sheep, had been shown to increase blood pressure by day 5 (Fig. 1, Group B) (8). This has now been confirmed in an additional six experiments.

HYPERTENSINOGENIC STEROIDS IN ACTH HYPERTENSION

Of the many steroids recently identified in sheep adrenal vein blood during ACTH treatment, two compounds will increase blood pressure: 17α-hydroxy-progesterone (17α-OHP) and 17α,20α-dihydroxyprogesterone (17α,20α-diOHP). However, these had a hypertensive effect only if they were infused concurrently with the combined steroid infusion. These experiments will now be presented in more detail. Intravenous steroid infusion was carried out after a control period over 5 days, using the same protocol as with the ACTH (19) and the steroid infusion experiments (8).

17α-OHP

Five animals in the first group were given a combined steroid infusion together with 17α-OHP at 3 μmoles/hr = 1 mg/hr intravenously for 5 days. This rate approximated adrenal secretion measured during ACTH treatment. Systolic blood pressure increased from 82 $\pm$ 1 (SEM) to 94 $\pm$ 2 and 102 $\pm$ 2 mm Hg on the fourth and fifth day, respectively ($p < 0.05$, and $p < 0.005$) (Fig. 1, Group C). Diastolic pressure showed a significant increase from 56 $\pm$ 1 to 61 $\pm$ 1 mm Hg by day 2 ($p < 0.005$) and 74 $\pm$ 2 mm Hg by day 5 ($p < 0.005$). Neither systolic nor diastolic blood pressure was elevated within 24 hr.

17α,20α-diOHP

Six animals in this second group were given a combined steroid infusion together with 17α,20α-diOHP at 1.5 μmoles/hr = 500 μg/hr approximating the measured values during ACTH treatment. Systolic blood pressure was significantly elevated within 24 hr, rising from a control of 85 $\pm$ 2 to 92 $\pm$ 3 mm Hg ($p < 0.01$) (Fig. 1, Group D). On day 5 of infusion, systolic blood pressure was 100 $\pm$ 3 mm Hg. Diastolic blood pressure was also significantly elevated within the first 24 hr, rising from a control of 60 $\pm$ 3 to 68 $\pm$ 3 mm Hg ($p < 0.01$), and was further elevated on day 5 of infusion to 70 $\pm$ 2 mm Hg ($p < 0.005$). This increased blood pressure and other metabolic changes are virtually indistinguishable from those observed following ACTH treatment.

Infusion of 17α-OHP and 17α,20α-diOHP with Combined Steroid

When 17α-OHP and 17α,20α-diOHP were infused concurrently with the combined steroid mixture, the effect was similar to that with 17α,20α-diOHP and combined steroid infusion.

Comment

The mechanism by which ACTH and, in particular, 17α,20α-diOHP influence blood pressure remains obscure. From these studies, the fact that on their own they are incapable of increasing blood pressure and the fact that they did not reduce the salivary sodium/potassium ratio on ipsilateral carotid artery infusion in the sodium-deficient and adrenalectomized sheep do not suggest a classic mineralocorticoid action. It is unlikely that they act as glucocorticoids because doubling the cortisol infusion rate of the combined steroid infusion will not mimic the hypertensive effect of ACTH. If 17α,20α-diOHP is not a glucocorticoid, then recognition of a class of steroids that will increase blood pressure, acting in concert with other steroids and dependent on sodium availability, but that are not classic mineralocorticoids has important implications for future clinical research in other experimental models of hypertension. Of particular interest are the recent studies on three patients with glucocorticoid-suppressible hypertension (14,15,25); they suggest the existence of as yet uncharacterized adrenal steroids that are under ACTH control and that may elevate blood pressure.

SODIUM AND HYPERTENSION

A large body of data, both clinical and experimental, points to an intimate relationship between sodium and hypertension. The role of sodium in our model of hypertension was examined in four situations: (a) severe sodium subtraction following parotid duct cannulation prior to 5 days of ACTH treatment; (b) severe sodium subtraction during ACTH treatment; (c) bilateral nephrectomy before ACTH treatment; and (d) ACTH treatment following chronic low-salt intake.

Sodium Depletion Prior to ACTH Treatment

Sodium-Depletion Period

In a sodium-depletion period of 48 hr prior to ACTH (Fig. 2), the mean urinary and salivary sodium loss was 480 ± 46 mmoles ($n = 6$). There was no significant fall in blood pressure.

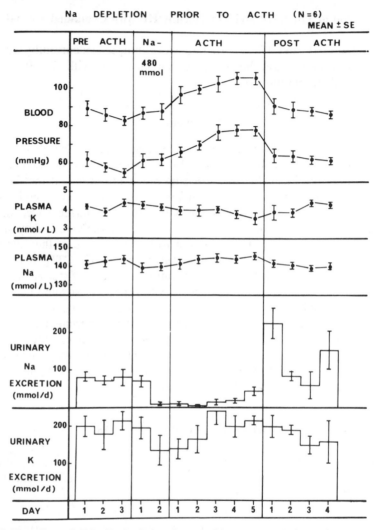

FIG. 2. The effect of 48-hr Na depletion, by parotid duct cannulation, prior to administration of ACTH on blood pressure, plasma [NA] and [K], and urinary Na and K excretion.

ACTH-Treatment Period

ACTH resulted in an increase in systolic blood pressure from 88 ± 4 to 97 ± 4 mm Hg within 24 hr ($p < 0.05$). Diastolic pressure also rose from 63 ± 3 to 66 ± 2 mm Hg ($p < 0.01$). By day 5 of ACTH treatment, blood pressure had risen to 106/78 mm Hg.

Sodium Depletion During ACTH Treatment

ACTH-Treatment Period

The ACTH-treatment period was extended from 5 to 7 days to accommodate the 2-day sodium depletion (Fig. 3). The effects of ACTH on blood pressure, plasma sodium potassium, urinary sodium, and potassium excretion are similar to those previously reported (19).

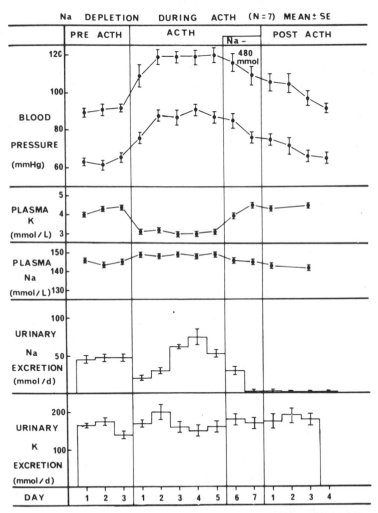

FIG. 3. The effect on blood pressure, plasma [Na] and [K], and urinary Na and K excretion of 48-hr Na depletion, by parotid duct cannulation, after 5-day administration of ACTH. ACTH was continued during the Na depletion.

Sodium-Depletion Period

With ACTH administration continuing, sodium depletion of 480 ± 43 mmoles ($n = 7$) over a 48-hr period resulted in a fall of systolic blood pressure from 120 ± 4 to 109 ± 5 mm Hg ($p < 0.05$). This value is still markedly elevated when compared to the pretreatment level of 92 ± 5 mm Hg ($p < 0.01$). Similarly, for diastolic pressure, sodium depletion resulted in a drop from 87 ± 3 to 76 ± 3 mm Hg ($p < 0.01$), but this was still greater than the pre-ACTH value of 66 ± 2 mm Hg ($p < 0.05$).

Bilateral Nephrectomy Before ACTH Treatment

ACTH was given 24 hr after bilateral nephrectomy. Blood pressure response was not different from the intact animal with ACTH administration over 3 to 5 days ($n = 5$).

ACTH Treatment Following Chronic Low-Salt Diet

Sodium Intake Less than 5 mmoles/Day

Sheep ($n = 3$) previously fed for some weeks on all grain rations of low sodium and potassium content did not become hypertensive following 5 days of ACTH treatment. Control blood pressure was 85/61 mm Hg and 90/68 mm Hg on day 1 and 90/67 mm Hg on day 5.

Sodium Intake of 10 mmoles/Day

Animals in this series had rumen cannulae surgically inserted. An additional daily electrolyte supplement of 10 mmoles of sodium and 100 mmoles of potassium was infused. In this group ($n = 3$), the blood pressure rose from 80/58 to 101/75 mm Hg by day 5.

Implications

(a) Acute sodium depletion (20 to 25% of exchangeable sodium) prior to ACTH does not modify hypertension.

(b) Acute sodium depletion (20 to 25% of exchangeable sodium) during ACTH does not return blood pressure to normal.

(c) The blood pressure response need not be associated with any change of external sodium balance.

(d) It appears likely, from preliminary data, that further chronic studies on low-salt intake will demonstrate a permissive role for sodium in the development of hypertension.

ACKNOWLEDGMENTS

This research was supported by the National Health and Medical Research Council of Australia, the Laura Bushell Trust, the National Heart Foundation of Australia, and G. D. Searle & Co.

REFERENCES

1. Adlin, E. V., Channick, B. T., and Marks, A. D. (1969): Salivary sodium-potassium ratio and plasma renin activity in hypertension. *Circulation,* 39:685.
2. Brown, J. J., Davies, D. L., Lever, A. F., and Robertson, J. I. S. (1964): Variations in plasma renin concentration in physiological and pathological states. *Can. Med. Assoc. J.,* 90:201.
3. Carey, R. M., Douglas, J. G., Schweikert, J. R., and Liddle, G. W. (1972): The syndrome of essential hypertension and suppressed plasma renin activity. *Arch. Intern. Med.,* 130:849.
4. Crane, M. G., Harris, J. J., and Johns, V. J. (1972): Hyporeninemic hypertension. *Am. J. Med.,* 52:457.
5. Dahl, L. K., Heine, M., and Tassinari, L. (1963): High salt content of Western infants diet: Possible relationship to hypertension in the adult. *Nature,* 198:1204.
6. Denton, D. A. (1973): Sodium and hypertension. In: *Proc. Int. Workshop Conference,* edited by M. P. Sambhi, pp. 46–54. Excerpta Medica, Amsterdam.
7. Denton, D. A. (1973): The brain and sodium homeostasis. *Conditional Reflex,* 8:125.
8. Fan, J. S. K., Coghlan, J. P., Denton, D. A., Oddie, C. J., Scoggins, B. A., and Shulkes, A. A. (1975): The effect of intravenous infusion of corticosteroids on blood pressure, electrolytes and water metabolism in sheep. *Am. J. Physiol.,* 228:1695.
9. Gunnels, J. C., McGuffin, W. L., Robinson, R. R., Grim, C. E., Wells, S., Silver, D., and Glenn, J. F. (1970): Hypertension, adrenal abnormalities, and alterations in plasma renin activity. *Ann. Intern. Med.,* 73:901.
10. Helmer, O. M. (1964): Renin activity in blood from patients with hypertension. *Can. Med. Assoc. J.,* 90:221.
11. Jose, A., Crout, J. R., and Kaplan, N. M. (1970): Suppressed plasma renin activity in essential hypertension. *Ann. Intern. Med.,* 72:9.
12. Melby, J. C., Dale, S. L., Grekin, R. J., Gaunt, R., and Wilson, T. E. (1972): 18-Hydroxy-11 deoxycorticosterone (18-OH-DOC) secretion in experimental and human hypertension. *Recent Prog. Horm. Res.,* 28:287.
13. Neusser, E. (1897): Die Erkrankungen der Nebennieren. In: *Specielle pathologie und Therapie,* Vol. 18, p. 71. Holder, Vienna.
14. New, M. I., Saenger, P. H., Levine, L. S., and Peterson, R. E. (1975): New evidence for a steroid hormone capable of producing hypertension in man. *Bull. N.Y. Acad. Med.,* 51:1180.
15. New, M. I., Saenger, P. H., Peterson, R. E., and Ulick, S. (1975): Evidence for an ACTH stimulable hormone causing hypertension. *Bull. N.Y. Acad. Med.,* 51:1179.
16. Oliver, W. J., Cohen, E. L., and Neel, J. V. (1975): Blood pressure, sodium intake, and sodium related hormones in the Yanomamo Indians, a "no-salt" culture. *Circulation,* 52:146.
17. Oliver, I. T., Frei, P., Levy, S., and Bartova, A. (1975): Changes in the blood pressure, ECG and serum constituents induced by implantation of mineralocorticoids in intact dogs. In: *Programs and Abstracts, 57th Annual Meeting of the Endocrine Society,* New York, p. 301.
18. Oppenheimer, B. S., and Fishberg, A. M. (1924): The association of hypertension with suprarenal tumors. *Arch. Intern. Med.,* 34:631.
19. Scoggins, B. A., Coghlan, J. P., Denton, D. A., Fan, S. K., McDougall, J. G., Oddie, C. J., and Shulkes, A. A. (1974): The metabolic effects of ACTH in the sheep. *Am. J. Physiol.,* 226:198.
20. Scoggins, B. A., Coghlan, J. P., Denton, D. A., Fan, J. S. K., McDougall, J. G., Oddie, C. J., and Shulkes, A. A. (1975): The role of adrenocortical hormones in ACTH induced hypertension. *J. Clin. Exp. Pharmacol. Physiol.,* 2:119.

21. Sennett, J. A., Brown, R. D., Island, D. P., Yarbo, L. R., Watson, J. T., Slaton, P. E., Hollifield, J. W., and Liddle, G. W. (1975): Evidence for a new mineralocorticoid in patients with low-renin essential hypertension. *Circ. Res., 36*(Suppl. 1):2.
22. Shulkes, A. A., Coghlan, J. P., Denton, D. A., Fan, J. S. K., Robinson, P. M., and Scoggins, B. A. (1974): The effect of adrenal denervation on ACTH induced hypertension in sheep. *J. Clin. Exp. Pharmacol. Physiol., 1*:479.
23. Sinnett, P. F., and Whyte, H. M. (1973): Epidemiological studies in a total highland population, Tukisenta, New Guinea. Cardiovascular disease and relevant clinical, electrocardiographic, radiological and biochemical findings. *J. Chronic Dis., 26*:256.
24. Spark, R. F., and Melby, J. C. (1971): Hypertension and low plasma renin activity: Presumptive evidence for mineralocorticoid excess. *Ann. Intern. Med., 75*:831.
25. Stockigt, J. R., Cukier, E. R., Higgs, E. J., Coghlan, J. P., Oddie, C. J., and Scoggins, B. A. (1975): Glucocorticoid-remediable mineralocorticoid hypertension. In: *Proceedings of the 18th Meeting of the Australian Endocrine Society.*
26. Vaughan, E. D., Laragh, J. H., Gavras, I., Buhler, F. R., Gavras, H., Brunner, H., and Baer, L. (1973): Volume factor in low and normal renin essential hypertension. Treatment with either spironolactone or chlorthalidone. *Am. J. Cardiol., 32*:523.
27. Woods, J. W., Liddle, G. W., Stant, E. G., Michelakis, A. M., and Brill, A. B. (1969): Effect of an adrenal inhibitor in hypertensive patients with suppressed renin. *Arch. Intern. Med., 123*:366.

Juvenile Hypertension, edited by
M. I. New and L. S. Levine. Raven
Press, New York © 1977.

Hypertension in the Young Rat

John P. Rapp

*Departments of Medicine and Pathology, Medical College of Ohio,
Toledo, Ohio 43614*

This chapter reviews three models for hypertension in young rats: (a) adrenal regeneration hypertension, (b) genetic hypertension, and very briefly, (c) teratogenic hypertension.

Adrenal regeneration hypertension is produced by removing one adrenal and enucleating the other, taking care to leave the capsule and its blood supply intact. The enucleated gland regenerates a new adrenal cortex without a medulla. There is a blood pressure rise associated with this regeneration, and it is more dramatic if the rats are unilaterally nephrectomized and given 1% saline to drink. Brownie et al. (7) have shown that the blood pressure rise in response to adrenal regeneration is more rapid and reaches higher levels if the enucleation procedure is initiated in weanling rats as compared to rats 4 to 5 months old (Fig. 1).

Adrenal regeneration hypertension is caused by the excess secretion of deoxycorticosterone (DOC) by the regenerating adrenal (1,6,8,32). This excess DOC production is transient, reaching a peak at about 3 to 4 weeks after enucleation and returning to normal with completed regeneration (6,8). Concomitant with the rise in blood pressure, there is a marked shift of sodium into and potassium out of skeletal muscle cells; these electrolyte shifts correlate extremely well with blood pressure (31). The relationship between skeletal muscle potassium and blood pressure with adrenal regeneration is shown in Fig. 2. Of particular interest in Fig. 2 is the fact that the changes in the blood pressure of unilaterally nephrectomized, young, growing controls fed saline or water also correlate well with muscle potassium loss, so that all experimental groups fall along the same line. That is, the small increase in blood pressure in controls resembles a mild mineralocorticoid effect.

If there is high sensitivity to adrenal regeneration in young rats, the existing data do not explain whether this is caused by higher plasma DOC levels produced by younger rats with adrenal regeneration or by higher sensitivity of younger rats to comparable plasma DOC levels. Injections of DOC acetate are

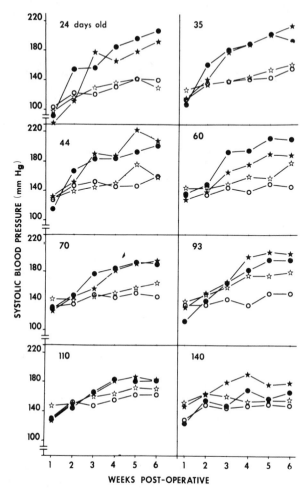

FIG. 1. Blood pressure response in rats to the adrenal regeneration procedure initiated at various ages. *Open symbols,* controls (unilateral nephrectomy, drinking 1% saline); *solid symbols,* adrenal regeneration rats (unilateral adrenalectomy, contralateral adrenal enucleation, unilateral nephrectomy, drinking 1% saline); *star,* male; *circle,* female. (From Brownie et al., ref. 7, with permission.)

more effective in increasing saline drunk and in producing hypertension and renal hypertrophy in young compared to mature rats (26). Since, in this experiment, the plasma DOC levels achieved by injection of the two age groups are also unknown, one cannot be certain if younger rats are more sensitive to DOC, or, for example, animals of various ages metabolize DOC or DOC acetate differently. In spite of these reservations, the data do suggest that young rats are metabolically poised for greater response to mineralocorticoid stimuli than older animals. The high muscle potassium of the younger animals and its loss with growth also appears to be a reflection of this metabolic state.

Dahl et al. (14) have developed two strains of rats by selective breeding. One strain is highly sensitive (S-strain) to the hypertensive effect of high-salt diet and the other is highly resistant (R-strain) to the hypertensive effect of salt. The blood pressure response to salt as a function of age was studied by Dahl et al. (17) in the S-strain. In this study, rats were fed 8% NaCl diet starting at ages 3 weeks (weanlings), 3 months, and 6 months. The results in Fig. 3 show that the blood pressure response to salt started at 3 weeks of age was more rapid and reached higher levels than that attained when salt was started after 3 months of age. Clearly, in these salt-sensitive rats, young animals are more sensitive to salt hypertension than older ones. Experience with the salt-susceptible rats has prompted Dahl (11) to seriously question the practice of adding salt to human baby food. In fact, it was possible to induce severe hypertension and death in the salt-susceptible rats by merely raising them on processed baby food (13).

What is known about the mechanisms of blood pressure control in the S- and R-strains? First, it has been shown that the inheritance of blood pressure in these models is polygenic, involving approximately two to four autosomal loci (25). One of these loci has been definitively identified and involves the

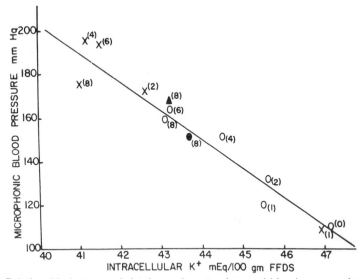

FIG. 2. Relationship between skeletal muscle potassium and blood pressure in adrenal regeneration and control rats. *X*, unilateral nephrectomy and adrenalectomy, contralateral adrenal enucleation, drinking 1% saline; *0*, unilateral nephrectomy, drinking 1% saline; ▲, unilateral nephrectomy and adrenalectomy, contralateral adrenal enucleation, drinking tap water; •, unilateral nephrectomy drinking water; *numbers in parentheses,* week of sacrifice after operation. The zero week point is from untreated intact controls aged 4 weeks.

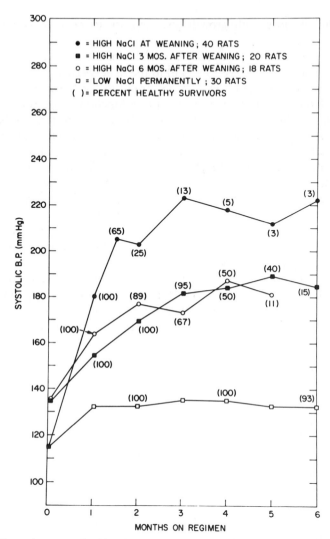

FIG. 3. Effect of age on the blood pressure response of the salt-susceptible Dahl rats to 8% salt diet. Control rats were fed low-salt (0.5% NaCl) diet from weaning and high-salt diet groups were started either at weaning (3 weeks of age) or at 3 or 6 months of age. (From Dahl et al., ref. 17, with permission.)

mutation of a cytochrome P-450 involved in adrenal steroid hydroxylation at positions 18 and 11β (33,34,36). This locus has two alleles inherited by Mendelian co-dominance and results in increased secretion and increased blood levels of the weak mineralocorticoid 18-hydroxy-11-deoxycorticosterone (33,34). Genetic experiments show that this locus accounts for only 16% of the blood pressure difference between strains, and that the remaining 84% must be caused by the other loci (34). One of these "other loci" involves the

'lase (DBH) activity in serum, adrenals, and mesenteric vessels is in-
over the control strain at 3 weeks of age (27,28). This difference pre-
ypertension, but the difference disappears from serum by 6 weeks of age
3H is the enzyme for conversion of dopamine to norepinephrine. Its
serum could be a reflection of sympathetic nerve activity, although this
iversally accepted. In fact, adult SH rats have normal serum DBH but
:d (sympathetic) splanchnic nerve activity (30). At this point, it is quite
ble to accept the early, transient increase in serum and tissue DBH as
ve of an important, but poorly understood, neural mechanism for the
ment of the variety of genetic hypertension existent in SH rats.
:t al. (37) found that with blood samples obtained from anesthetized
: Japanese SH rats show a transient rise in plasma and renal renin
occurring at 3 to 6 weeks of age, and that plasma renin then decreases
:reasing blood pressure. Campbell (9) indicates that this elevation in
renin in young SH rats is readily demonstrated in samples from
tized rats, but is not seen in samples from unanesthetized (decapitated)
us, the young Japanese SH rats do seem to show an exaggerated renin
in response to anesthesia. Sinaiko and Mirkin (38) reported that renal
as also transiently increased in the SH rat, but the age group studied
from the fetal rat to 3 weeks of age; therefore, this study does not
in ages with those of Sen et al. and Campbell. Another study on renin
g rats was performed by Bianchi et al. (2), who found that plasma renin
1HS was lower than that in the control strain. It is unclear whether the
ansient increase in plasma renin in Japanese SH rats in response to
sia is related to the transient rise in plasma DBH seen in this strain.
e renin is released by neurogenic mechanisms (see ref. 18 for review),
isient increase in both DBH and plasma renin activity response to
sia might be a reflection of the same underlying neurogenic aberration.
rficially, at least, it appears that of the four rat genetic models on which
; much physiological evidence, two have a renal, salt, and water
ism of importance (i.e., Dahl's S-strain and Bianchi's MHS rats) and
'e a significant neural mechanism (i.e., New Zealand GH and Japanese
). Whether this distinction is real or whether workers with each strain
st pursued different lines of thought is impossible to tell without, for
e, data on the nervous system in S-strain and MHS, or data on renal
antation from SH and GH rats.
man and White (22) produced hypertension in weanling rats and dogs
ing them on diets deficient in either potassium or choline for 21 days.
procedures evidently resulted in renal lesions and, as such, may
nt a well-known response to reduction in renal function. In another
Grollman and Grollman (21) reported that when pregnant rats were
arious treatments, the offspring became hypertensive at 1 year old.
ents that resulted in hypertensive offspring were administration of
one, DOC, cortisone, progesterone, chlorothiazide (presumably via

pituitary gland, which in R-rats accumulates lai
colloid in the pituitary cleft. This colloid contains
unique for R-rats, and genetic experiments indicate
tion is associated with up to 40% of the blood pre
and R-strains (35). The function of this protein is co
part of the remaining blood pressure difference bet
ultimately be accounted for by the kidney. It hi
transplantation between S- and R-rats, that an S-ki
salt sensitivity and that an R-kidney protects agains
The specific mechanisms are, however, unknown.

Data are available for the blood pressure in y
genetically hypertensive strains. In both the sp
(SH) rats of Okamoto and Aoki (29) and the Milan
of Bianchi et al. (5), the blood pressure is not ele
matched control rats at weaning, but the blood pres
growth and is first significantly higher than controls
the New Zealand genetically hypertensive (GH) rats
is significantly higher than in the control strain, eve
any case, genetically hypertensive rats of any of
pathologically rising blood pressures well before m
models for hypertension, immature animals with
pressure develop severe hypertension with growth a
that a genetically mediated high blood pressure at a y
future disease in the rat. This should be no less tru

There are other interesting data in young animals f
sive rat strains. Bianchi et al. (2) have shown that MH
than normotensive rats (NR) during growth (24 to 66
MHS rats, urine output and fluid consumption are tr
suggests that the MHS develops hypertension because
and water metabolism of the kidney. Bianchi et al. (
cross transplantation of kidneys between MHS and
hypertension in the MHS was related to the kidney.

Thus, the data suggest that in both Dahl's S-rats an
kidney is intimately involved in the hypertensive p
indirectly by being the affector organ for hormonal
data from two other genetically hypertensive rat strai
factors for hypertension operate through the nervou
both in the Japanese SH and in the New Zealand GH n
development of the sympathetic nervous system in no
sympathectomy or by treatment with 6-hydroxydopar
development of hypertension during growth (10,19
pharmacological blockade of the sympathetic nerv
methonium in New Zealand GH rats also suggests an
ponent for the hypertension (39). In the Japanese

potassium deficiency), low-potassium diet, high-sodium diet, or choline-deficient diet. In addition, Grollman and Grollman stated that no renal lesions were present in these hypertensive offspring, although these treatments would be expected to produce such lesions. This is, nevertheless, provocative work worthy of further study.

SUMMARY

There is evidence suggesting that young rats are more sensitive than older ones to the hypertensive effect of mineralocorticoids plus salt, or the hypertensive effect of salt alone.

There are four well-known strains of rats that have been selectively bred for hypertension. Young rats from these strains show increased blood pressure well before maturity. In two of these strains (Dahl's salt-sensitive and Bianchi's MHS), the evidence indicates that the hypertension is caused by aberrations of salt and water metabolism with intimate involvement of the kidney. In the other two (Okamoto and Aoki's Japanese SH and Smirk's New Zealand GH rats), a strong neurogenic component to the hypertension is indicated.

There is also suggestive evidence that treatments applied to pregnant rats, such as steroids or dietary regimens that can cause hypertension, result in hypertensive offspring.

REFERENCES

1. Bergon, L., Gallant, S., and Brownie, A. C. (1975): Serum 11-deoxycorticosterone levels in adrenal-regeneration hypertension under conditions of quiescence and stress. *Steroids,* 25:323–342.
2. Bianchi, G., Baer, P. G., Fox, U., Dazzi, L., Pagetti, D., and Giovannetti, H. M. (1975): Changes in renin, water balance and sodium balance during development of high blood pressure in genetically hypertensive rats. *Circ. Res.,* 36,37(Suppl. I):I-153–I-161.
3. Bianchi, G., Fox, U., Di Francesco, G. F., Bardi, U., and Radice, M., (1973): Hypertensive role of the kidney in spontaneously hypertensive rats. *Clin. Sci. Molec. Med.,* 45:135S–139S.
4. Bianchi, G., Fox, U., Di Francesco, G. F., Giovannetti, A. M., and Pagetti, D. (1974): Blood pressure changes produced by kidney cross-transplantation between hypertensive rats and normotensive rats. *Clin. Sci. Molec. Med.,* 47:435–448.
5. Bianchi, G., Fox, U., and ImPasciati, E. (1974): The development of a new strain of spontaneously hypertensive rats. *Life Sci.,* 14:339–347.
6. Brown, R. D., Gaunt, R., Gisoldi, E., and Smith, H. (1972): The role of deoxycorticosterone in adrenal regeneration hypertension. *Endocrinology,* 91:921–924.
7. Brownie, A. C., Bernardis, L. L., Miwa, T., Kamura, S., and Skelton, F. R. (1966): The influence of age and sex on the development of adrenal regeneration hypertension. *Lab. Invest.,* 15:1342–1356.
8. Brownie, A. C., and Skelton, F. R. (1965): The metabolism of progesterone-4-^{14}C by adrenal homogenates from rats with adrenal regeneration hypertension. *Steroids,* 6:47–68.
9. Campbell, W. B. (1974): Renin in the spontaneously hypertensive rat. (Letter to the editor.) *Circ. Res.,* 35:961–962.
10. Clark, D. W. J. (1971): Effects of immunosympathectomy on development of high blood pressure in genetically hypertensive rats. *Circ. Res.,* 28:330–336.
11. Dahl, L. K. (1968): Salt in processed baby foods. *Am. J. Clin. Nutr.* 21:787–792.

12. Dahl, L. K., and Heine, M. (1975): Primary role of renal homografts in setting chronic blood pressure levels in rats. *Circ. Res.,* 36:692–696.
13. Dahl, L. K., Heine, M., Leitl, G., and Tassinari, L. (1970): Hypertension and death from consumption of processed baby foods by rats. *Proc. Soc. Exp. Biol. Med.,* 133:1405–1408.
14. Dahl, L., Heine, M., and Tassinari, L. (1962): Effects of chronic excess salt ingestion. Evidence that genetic factors play an important role in susceptibility to experimental hypertension. *J. Exp. Med.,* 115:1173–1190.
15. Dahl, L. K., Heine, M., and Thompson, K. (1972): Genetic influence of renal homografts on the blood pressure of rats from different strains. *Proc. Soc. Exp. Biol. Med.,* 140:852–856.
16. Dahl, L. K., Heine, M., and Thompson, K. (1974): Genetic influence of the kidneys on blood pressure. Evidence from renal homografts in rats with opposite predispositions to hypertension. *Circ. Res.,* 34:94–101.
17. Dahl, L. K., Knudsen, K. D., Heine, M. A., and Leitl, G. J. (1968): Effects of chronic excess salt ingestion. Modification of experimental hypertension in the rat by variations in the diet. *Circ. Res.,* 22:11–18.
18. Davis, J. O. (1971): What signals the kidney to release renin? *Circ. Res.,* 28:301–306.
19. Finch, L., Cohen, M., Horst, W. D. (1973): Effects of 6-hydroxydopamine at birth on the development of hypertension in the rat. *Life Sci.,* 13:1403–1410.
20. Folkow, B., Hallback, M., Lundgren, Y., and Weiss, L. (1972): The effects of immunosympathectomy on blood pressure and vascular reactivity in normal and spontaneously hypertensive rats. *Acta Physiol. Scand.,* 84:512–523.
21. Grollman, A., and Grollman, E. F. (1962): The teratogenic induction of hypertension. *J. Clin. Invest.* 41:710–714.
22. Grollman, A., and White, F. H. (1958): Induction of renal hypertension in rats and dogs by potassium or choline deficiency. *Am. J. Physiol.,* 193:144–146.
23. Haeusler, G., Finch, L., and Thoenen, H. (1972): Central adrenergic neurones and the initiation and development of experimental hypertension. *Experientia,* 28:1200–1203.
24. Jones, D. R., and Dowd, D. A. (1970): Development of elevated blood pressure in young genetically hypertensive rats. *Life Sci.* 9(1):247–250.
25. Knudsen, K. D., Dahl, L. K., Thompson, K., Iwai, J., Heine, M., and Leitl, G. (1970): Effects of chronic excess salt ingestion. Inheritance of hypertension in the rat. *J. Exp. Med.,* 132:976–1000.
26. Musilova, H., Jelinek, J., and Albrecht, I. (1966): The age factor in experimental hypertension of the DCA type in rats. *Physiol. Bohemoslov.,* 15:525–531.
27. Nagatsu, T., Ikuta, K., Numata, Y., Kato, T., Sano, M., Nagatsu, I., Umezawa, H., Matsuzaki, M., and Takeuchi, T. (1976): Vascular and brain dopamine β-hydroxylase activity in young spontaneously hypertensive rats. *Science,* 191:290–291.
28. Nagatsu, T., Kato, T., Numata, Y., Ikuta, K., Umezawa, H., Matsuzaki, M., and Takeuchi, T. (1974): Serum dopamine β-hydroxylase activity in developing hypertensive rats. *Nature,* 251:630–631.
29. Okamoto, K., and Aoki, K. (1963): Development of a strain of spontaneously hypertensive rats. *Jpn. Circ. J.,* 27:282–293.
30. Okamoto, K., Nosaka, S., Yamori, Y., Matsumoto, M. (1967): Participation of neural factor in the pathogenesis of hypertension in the spontaneously hypertensive rat. *Jpn. Heart J.,* 8:168–180.
31. Rapp, J. P. (1964): Electrolyte and juxtaglomerular changes in adrenal regeneration hypertension. *Am. J. Physiol.,* 206:93–104.
32. Rapp, J. P. (1969): Deoxycorticosterone production in adrenal regeneration: *In vitro* vs. *in vivo* comparison. *Endocrinology,* 84:1409–1420.
33. Rapp, J. P., and Dahl, L. K. (1971): Adrenal steroidogenesis in rats bred for susceptibility and resistance to the hypertensive effect of salt. *Endocrinology,* 88:52–65.
34. Rapp, J. P., and Dahl, L. K. (1972): Mendelian inheritance of 18- and 11β-steroid hydroxylase activities in the adrenals of rats genetically susceptible or resistant to hypertension. *Endocrinology,* 90:1435–1446.
35. Rapp, J. P., and Dahl, L. K. (1974): Anatomical and protein electrophoretic observations on pituitary cleft colloid in rats genetically susceptible or resistant to salt hypertension. *Lab. Invest.,* 30:417–426.

36. Rapp, J. P., and Dahl, L. K. (1976): Mutant forms of cytochrome P-450 controlling both 18- and 11β-steroid hydroxylation in the rat. *Biochemistry,* 15:1235–1242.
37. Sen, S., Smeby, R. R., Bumpus, F. M. (1972): Renin in rats with spontaneous hypertension. *Circ. Res.,* 31:878–880.
38. Sinaiko, A., and Mirkin, B. L. (1974): Ontogenesis of the renin angiotensin system in spontaneously hypertensive and normal Wistar rats. *Circ. Res.,* 34:693–696.
39. Smirk, F. H. (1970): The neurogenically maintained component in hypertension. *Circ. Res.,* 26,27(Suppl. II):II-55–II-63.

Juvenile Hypertension, edited by
M. I. New and L. S. Levine. Raven
Press, New York © 1977.

Developmental Aspects of Renin Release and Sensitivity to Adrenergic Stimulation in Spontaneously Hypertensive Rats

M. H. Weinberger and *W. Aoi

Department of Medicine, Specialized Center of Research in Hypertension, Indiana University School of Medicine, Indianapolis, Indiana 46202

The spontaneously hypertensive rat (SHR) has been extensively studied as a model of idiopathic hypertension in man. Several studies have reported conflicting observations regarding renin activity in these animals (7,10,11). However, the study designs and their methods were dissimilar. In addition, studies of renin activity *in vivo* can be influenced by anesthetics, adrenergic factors, humoral agents, and hemodynamic changes (4). To examine factors directly influencing renin release, it has proved advantageous to employ an isolated *in vivo* system (1). Such a system is potentially informative in the study of basal levels of renin release as well as the response of renin to specific agents. Recent reports have suggested that hyperactivity of the sympathetic nervous system may be involved in the development and/or maintenance of hypertension in the SHR (5,8).

The present study was performed to examine developmental changes in renin release in the SHR, utilizing the isolated rat kidney slice system, and to compare such observations with those of normotensive rats of both Sprague-Dawley and Kyoto-Wistar strains. In addition, the sensitivity of renin release to norepinephrine was examined in kidney slices of SHR and Kyoto-Wistar rats of different ages.

MATERIALS AND METHODS

The techniques used in these studies have been previously reported (1). In brief, the kidneys are removed and two 0.5 mm slices are prepared from the

---

*Present address: Third Department of Medicine, Nagasaki University School of Medicine, 7-1 Sakamoto, Nagasaki City, Machi, Japan.

superficial cortex of each kidney with a Stadie-Riggs microtome. After washing in Robinsons' media, these slices are incubated at 25°C in a shaker saturated with 95% O_2 to 5% CO_2, for four successive 20-min periods. Renin release is stable for the four incubation periods (1), thus permitting each slice to serve as its own control. The second incubation period was utilized for measurement of basal renin release, and the third period, bracketed by control incubations (second and fourth periods), was utilized for the norepinephrine studies. After each period, media was aspirated and fresh media added. To measure renin activity, 0.05 ml of the renin-containing media from the kidney slice incubation was added to 2.5 nmoles hog renin substrate (Pentex Division, Miles Lab., Inc.); angiotensinase and converting enzyme inhibitors were also added and the mixture incubated at 37°C for 1 hr. The angiotensin I thus generated was quantified by radioimmunoassay. Appropriate blanks were subtracted and the results expressed as angiotensin I ng/mg dry kidney weight. Statistical analyses were performed by the paired t-test (for norepinephrine responses) and by the unpaired t-test for differences between animals. The relationship between age and basal renin release was analyzed by the linear regression technique.

RESULTS

The relationship between basal renin release and age for all three strains is shown in Fig. 1. Among Sprague-Dawley rats, a significant inverse linear relationship ($p < 0.001$) was observed from 1½ to 3 months of age. A similar relationship was observed ($p < 0.001$) in the SHR from 1½ to 4 months of age. In contrast, observations in the Kyoto-Wistar strain failed to show a decline in basal renin release with age. When basal renin release was compared among strains, there were no significant differences at 1½ and 2 months of age, but when observations from 3- to 7-month-old SHR were compared to age-matched Kyoto-Wistar controls, significant differences ($p < 0.05$ to < 0.001) were seen.

Figure 2 depicts the response of renin release to 1.5×10^{-9} M norepinephrine in kidney slices from SHR and Kyoto-Wistar strains at various ages. At every point, the addition of norepinephrine stimulated renin release significantly when compared to the preceding control period ($p < 0.05$). The magnitude of mean stimulation of renin release was consistently greater in kidney slices from the SHR than those from the Kyoto-Wistar controls at every age. However, as indicated in Fig. 2, the statistical significance of this increased response was not apparent in 1½ and 2-month-old animals.

DISCUSSION

The role of renin in the development and maintenance of hypertension in the SHR, an experimental model of idiopathic hypertension, is controversial.

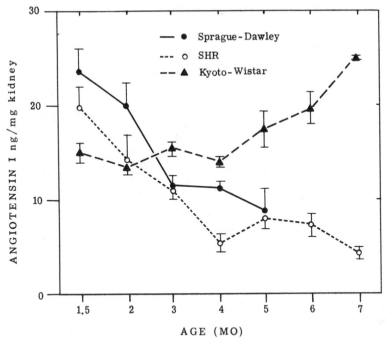

FIG. 1. Relationship between basal renin release and age in kidney slices from three strains of rats. Each point represents the mean of four slices from four animals; the bars are ± 1 SE. (From Aoi and Weinberger, ref. 2.)

A variety of reports have indicated that renin activity is increased (7), normal (6), or decreased (3, 10, 11) in SHR when compared to normotensive control animals. The possible explanations for these conflicting results are: (a) the ages of the animals studied; (b) the control strain used; (c) differing techniques of anesthesia and blood collection; and (d) differing techniques for measuring the renin system.

In the present study, an attempt was made to examine basal renin release from kidney slices. This system has the advantage of not being affected by a variety of hemodynamic and humoral factors that may influence renin release *in vivo*. In addition, developmental differences in renin release were examined, using the isolated *in vitro* system. The results of the present study show a linear decline in basal renin release with age in kidney slices from both SHR and Sprague-Dawley rats that is absent in Kyoto-Wistar rats. This observation does not appear to be caused by elevation of blood pressure, at least in the Sprague-Dawley rats, because they remained normotensive. The observations of an age-related decline in renin release among SHR and Sprague-Dawley rats are similar to those reported for normotensive man (9). It is not clear why this decline was not seen in Kyoto-Wistar rats.

If the observations of basal renin release from kidney slices *in vitro* bear a

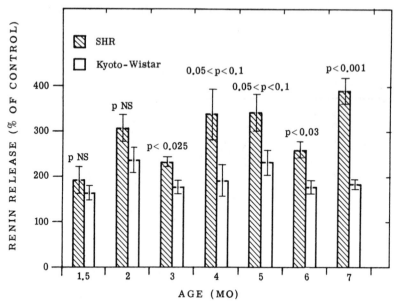

FIG. 2 Stimulation of renin release by norepinephrine in SHR and Kyoto-Wistar rats of varying age. Each bar represents the mean of four slices from four animals; the bars are ± 1 SE. Significance values presented represent the difference in responses between SHR and Kyoto-Wistar rats. (From Aoi and Weinberger, ref. 2.)

direct relationship to renin activity *in vivo,* then it becomes easier to reconcile some of the apparent contradictions reported regarding renin activity in the SHR. Renin release from the kidney slices was higher in 1½-month-old SHR than in Kyoto-Wistar, but when 3- to 7-month-old animals were studied significantly ($p < 0.05$ to $p < 0.001$), lower levels of basal renin release were seen in kidney slices from SHR. Thus, it can be anticipated that renin activity from young SHR might well be higher than that for Kyoto-Wistar controls and lower than that for older animals, as has been reported by other investigators (3,7,10,11). The relationship between these observations and the mechanism of hypertension cannot be discerned from the present study.

Because of recent reports suggesting that increased activity of the sympathetic nervous system may be involved in the pathophysiology of hypertension in the SHR (5, 8), the effect of norepinephrine on renin release was also studied in this isolated kidney slice system. The present study demonstrates an enhancement of sensitivity of renin release to norepinephrine in slices from the SHR. Furthermore, this enhanced sensitivity appears to increase with age in the SHR, whereas there is no discernible change in sensitivity with age in kidney slices from Kyoto-Wistar rats. Additional studies will be required to relate these observations to the level of sympathetic activity *in vivo.*

SUMMARY

Utilizing an isolated *in vitro* kidney slice system for the assessment of renin release, a developmental decline in renin release was observed in SHR and Sprague-Dawley rats but not in Kyoto-Wistar animals. In addition, while renin release is responsive to adrenergic stimulation in both SHR and Kyoto-Wistar strains, the magnitude of response is consistently greater in SHR, and increases with age. These studies confirm a suggested role for adrenergic stimulation in the pathophysiology of the hypertension in SHR.

ACKNOWLEDGMENTS

These studies were supported in part by grants from the USPHS, HL 14159, Specialized Center of Research in Hypertension (SCOR), and from the American Heart Association, Indiana Affiliate. The authors wish to express their gratitude to Ms. Gwendolyn Morgan for assistance in preparation of this manuscript and to Dr. David Henry for helpful advice in the conduct of these studies.

REFERENCES

1. Aoi, W., Wade, M. B., Rosner, D. R., and Weinberger, M. H. (1974): Renin release by rat kidney slices *in vitro:* Effects of cations and catecholamines. *Am. J. Physiol.,* 227:630–634.
2. Aoi, W., and Weinberger, M. H. (1976): The effect of age and norepinephrine on renin release by rat kidney slices in vitro. *Proc. Soc. Exp. Biol. Med.,* 151:47–52.
3. Baer, L., Knowlton, A., and Laragh, J. H. (1972): The role of sodium balance and the pituitary adrenal axis in the hypertension of spontaneously hypertensive rats. In: *Spontaneous Hypertension,* edited by K. Okamoto, pp. 203–209. Igaku Shoin, Tokyo.
4. Davis, J. O., and Freeman, R. H., (1976): Mechanisms regulating renin release. *Physiol. Rev.,* 56:1–56.
5. Folkow, B., Hallback, M., Lundgren, Y, and Weiss, L. (1970): Background of increased flow resistance and vascular reactivity in spontaneously hypertensive rats. *Acta Physiol. Scand.,* 80:93–106.
6. Forman, B. H., and Mulrow, P. J. (1974): Effect of propranolol on blood pressure and plasma renin activity in the spontaneously hypertensive rat. *Circ. Res.,* 35:215–221.
7. DeJong, W., Lovenberg, W., and Sjoerdsma, A. (1972): Increased plasma renin activity in the spontaneously hypertensive rat. *Proc. Soc. Exp. Biol. Med.,* 139:1213–1216.
8. Judy, W. V., Watanabe, A. M., Henry, D. P., Besch, H. R., Jr., Murphy, W. A., and Hockel, G. M. (1976): Sympathetic nerve activity: Role in regulation of blood pressure in the spontaneously hypertensive rat. *Circ. Res.,* 38(Suppl. II): 21–29.
9. Sambhi, M. P., Crane, M. G., and Genest, J. (1973): Essential hypertension: New concepts about mechanisms. *Ann. Intern. Med.,* 79:411–424.
10. Sen, S., Smeby, R. R., and Bumpus, F. M. (1972): Renin in rats with spontaneous hypertension. *Circ. Res.,* 31:876–880.
11. Sokabe, H. (1965): Renin-angiotensin system in the spontaneously hypertensive rat. *Nature,* 205:90.

Juvenile Hypertension, edited by
M. I. New and L. S. Levine. Raven
Press, New York © 1977.

Comment: Animal Models for Childhood Hypertension

Lenore S. Levine

These studies provide interesting data on the interplay of diet, genetics, and hormones in the development of animal hypertension. They suggest the multifactorial nature of hypertension in man and document the necessity and importance of studying these factors in the young. The young animal as a model for hypertension in childhood has not been investigated extensively, and may prove an important tool in hypertension research.

Dr. Edelman's comments on steroid receptors and hypertension are presented later in this volume.

Juvenile Hypertension, edited by
M. I. New and L. S. Levine. Raven
Press, New York © 1977.

Aldosterone in Childhood

A. Avinoam Kowarski and Claude J. Migeon

*The Harriet Lane Service, Children's Medical and Surgical Center, Johns Hopkins
University School of Medicine, Baltimore, Maryland 21205*

A single determination of the aldosterone concentration in blood is often of little use because of the wide fluctuations in hormone levels during the day (1). For this reason, the daily integrated concentration, which is the average concentration during a 24-hr period, may be a more useful determination. Since a decrease in the metabolic clearance rate (MCR) of aldosterone may occur in a significant percentage of individuals suffering from essential hypertension (2,3), an abnormally high integrated concentration of aldosterone may also occur while the secretion rate is within normal range. Consequently, it is important to determine not only the secretion rate but also the integrated concentration of aldosterone in the same individual. These two determinations should best be carried out simultaneously during the same day because they, as well as the MCR, do vary from 1 day to another.

A proper evaluation of the role of aldosterone in hypertension during childhood cannot be carried out prior to establishing the normal range for the aldosterone secretion rate and integrated concentration. This normal range must be established in healthy children, since the normal levels cannot be obtained from studies in adults. This chapter includes evidence that the aldosterone secretion rate during childhood, when corrected for body surface area, is significantly higher than that of adults. During the first year of life, the integrated concentration of aldosterone is also significantly higher than that of adults. During the first week of life, the plasma levels are similar to those of adults in a standing position but higher than those of supine adults. The human fetus maintains a higher concentration of aldosterone than its mother.

ALDOSTERONE SECRETION RATE DURING INFANCY AND CHILDHOOD

Children suffering from the salt-losing form of congenital adrenal hyperplasia require replacement therapy with mineralocorticoids. The appropriate dosage was established more than 25 years ago by trial and error (4). Newborn infants were found to require 1 to 2 mg i.m. deoxycorticosterone acetate daily. This dosage was surprisingly high because it is similar to that required by adults. The daily requirement for mineralocorticoid remains constant throughout life despite an increase in body weight from 3½ to 70 kg. These findings are in contrast with the glucocorticoid requirement that is closely related to body size, remaining 12 ± 3 mg/m²/24 hr throughout life (5,6). As shown in Fig. 1, the only exception is during the first week of life, when the cortisol secretion is 18 mg/m²/24 hr.

The aldosterone secretion rates of normal children are shown in Fig. 2; the values are not corrected for body size. It should be noted that during the first week of life, the aldosterone secretion rate was slightly below the normal range for adults. The other children, ranging in age from 2 to 12 weeks, had an aldosterone secretion rate that was within the normal range for normal adults. These observations agree with the high requirement for mineralocorticoids found in infants suffering from the salt-losing form of congenital adrenal hyperplasia. One could speculate that the lower aldosterone secretion values of the first week of life are related to the 10% weight loss that occurs after birth.

PLASMA ALDOSTERONE CONCENTRATIONS DURING INFANCY AND CHILDHOOD

The high aldosterone secretion rate found in children may be caused by either an end-organ insensitivity relative to that found in adults or a relatively

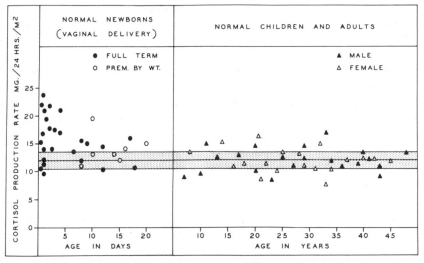

FIG. 1. Cortisol secretion rate, corrected for body surface area in normal newborn infants, children, and adults. (From Kowarski et al., ref. 1.)

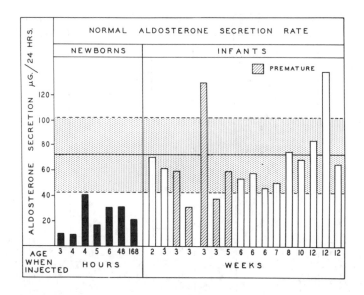

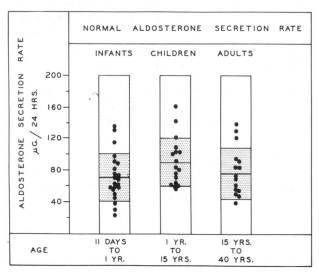

FIG. 2. Aldosterone secretion rates in normal infants less than 1 week of age compared to infants 2 to 12 weeks of age. *Bars,* secretion rate for one subject; *shaded area,* mean ± 1 SD for the 8-day to 12-month age group. (From Weldon et al., ref. 7.)

high MCR. In the first case, an increased aldosterone concentration should accompany the high secretion rate during early childhood. In the second case, the plasma aldosterone level should remain in the range of normal adults. Figure 3 presents the plasma aldosterone concentrations in normal subjects; the mean plasma aldosterone concentration obtained for the group 1 week to 1 year of age was significantly higher ($p < 0.005$) than that of all the other age

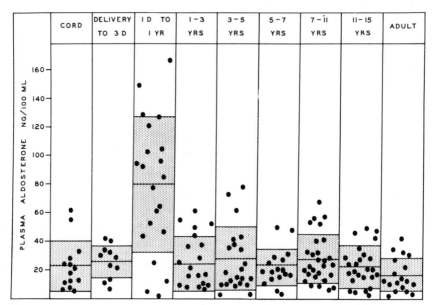

FIG. 3. Plasma aldosterone concentrations in normal subjects (*shaded area*, mean ± 1 SD for each group). The values for cord plasma and infants up to 3 days of age were determined in those subjects whose mothers had been maintained on a normal sodium diet throughout pregnancy. The mean obtained for the group 1 week to 1 year of age was significantly higher than that of all other age groups. (From Kowarski et al., ref. 8.)

groups. A single determination of the plasma aldosterone concentration in an individual reflects the situation at any particular time. Since the plasma aldosterone level fluctuates widely during the day (1), the dispersion of the results in each age group is caused by the combined effect of individual differences and the moment-to-moment fluctuations in the aldosterone concentration of each individual. The human fetus maintains slightly, but significantly, higher plasma aldosterone concentration than its mother and secretes part of its own aldosterone (Fig. 4).

MCR OF ALDOSTERONE AT VARIOUS AGES

As mentioned earlier, the plasma aldosterone levels are determined by the rate of secretion and removal from the circulation. Unfortunately, no direct measurement of the MCR in infants has been made. Using the mean plasma concentration and the secretion rates of 21 infants, the MCR of these infants was *estimated;* the results are presented in Table 1.

It must be pointed out that the aldosterone concentrations of our study were obtained from plasma samples collected at 8 to 9 a.m. Yet, we have reported (1) that the plasma level of aldosterone tends to be higher in the morning hours. As a result of this bias, the MCR of aldosterone in Table 1 is underestimated. In spite of this inherent error, the calculated value for the MCR in our

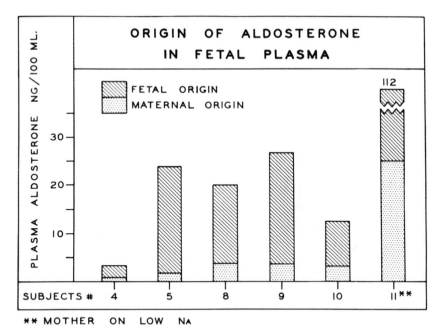

FIG. 4. Origin of aldosterone in fetal plasma. (From Beitins et al., ref. 11.)

three age groups can be used for the purpose of comparison. As seen in Table 1, the MCR of aldosterone, related to body surface area, is relatively similar in the three age groups, whereas the aldosterone secretion rate is higher in infancy. It can, therefore, be concluded that the increased aldosterone concentration during the first year of life is primarily attributable to an increased secretion in relation to body size.

FIRST SALT-LOSING CRISIS IN CONGENITAL ADRENAL HYPERPLASIA

Figure 5 describes the age at which 70 salt-losing infants had their first adrenal crisis. Twenty-four of the 70 patients had their initial crisis during the

TABLE 1. *Metabolic clearance rate of aldosterone—effect of age*

Age	MPA (ng/ 100 ml)	ASR (μg/24 hr)	ASR (μg/m²/24 hr)	"Estimated" MCR[a] (liters/24 hr)	"Estimated" MCR[a] (liters/m²/24 hr)
11 days–1 yr	79.9	72	312	90	390
1–15 yr	24.9	91	110	365	443
Adult	16.6	80	47	483	234

[a]Calculated from the mean values of aldosterone secretion rate (ASR) and the mean plasma aldosterone (MPA) concentration.

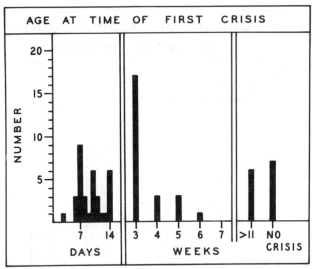

FIG. 5. The age at which the first salt-losing crisis occurred in the 70 patients with the salt-losing form of congenital adrenal hyperplasia. (From Kowarski et al., ref. 10.)

first 2 weeks of life, one at 3 days and all others at or after 6 days of age. It has been shown that the aldosterone secretion rate of these infants was extremely low (9). It appears that these infants, as well as normal newborns, can sustain salt and water loss during the first few days of life. After that time, the normal newborns increase their aldosterone secretion and, hence, maintain their homeostasis, whereas patients with adrenal hyperplasia are unable to do so and therefore develop an acute crisis. It is of interest to note that patients who developed their adrenal crisis later in life usually had a less severe defect and were able to secrete aldosterone (Fig. 6).

FLUCTUATIONS OF PLASMA ALDOSTERONE

The dramatic fluctuation in the plasma aldosterone level is shown in Fig. 7, which represents the results of a study using a portable nonthrombogenic blood withdrawal system. This system was used to monitor integrated concentration of aldosterone in an individual for a period of 2 days. The first study was carried out during normal activity and the second study during a day spent mostly in bed (1). Although the aldosterone levels fluctuated with no apparent pattern, the overall levels and 24-hr integrated concentrations were lower during the day spent mostly in a supine position than during the day of normal activity.

Some of the aldosterone peaks during the day may be related to quick ACTH release, perhaps because of "stress" conditions. This would be compatible with the finding that intravenous ACTH results in temporary elevation of plasma aldosterone levels (Fig. 8).

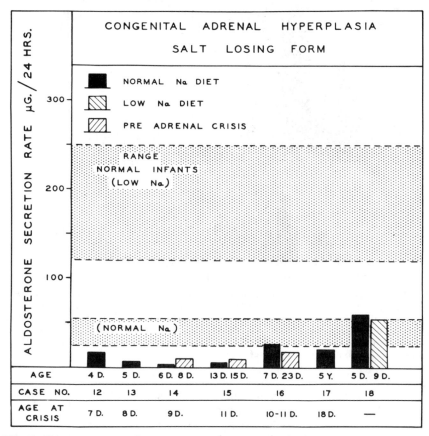

FIG. 6. Aldosterone secretion rate in patients with the salt-losing form of congenital adrenal hyperplasia. The seven patients presented in this figure had no therapy and were receiving a normal sodium diet at the time of the study. A second study was carried out on patients 14, 15, and 16 just before an adrenal crisis and on patient 18 when on a low-sodium diet. The patients are arranged according to the severity of their salt-losing tendency as determined by their age at the time of the first spontaneous adrenal crisis; patient 18 did not go into crisis even when put on a low-sodium diet for 4 days. (From Kowarski et al., ref. 9.)

Despite the erratic appearance of 24-hr aldosterone curves, the study of groups of subjects suggests a diurnal pattern of plasma aldosterone levels (1) somewhat similar to that of cortisol (Fig. 9).

EFFECTS OF SODIUM DEPLETION

It is well established that sodium depletion in adults results in increased aldosterone secretion (7). Figure 10 represents aldosterone concentration in cord and newborn plasma. The mothers had been either on normal or on low-sodium intake, with or without diuretics, before delivery. The results are

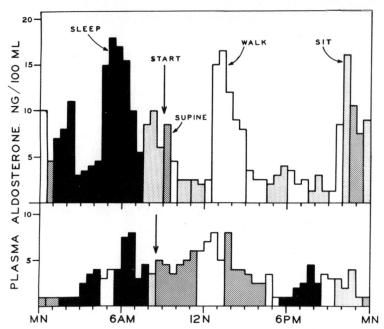

FIG. 7. Fluctuations of integrated concentration of plasma aldosterone in a normal subject. The study was carried out on two occasions: during normal activity and when in bed during most of the day. *Shaded areas,* body posture during each 30-min period; *black areas,* periods of sleep; *heavy shaded bars,* periods when the subject was awake but supine; *light-shaded bars,* periods when the subject was sitting; *white bars,* when subject was standing and walking. (From Kowarski et al., ref. 1.)

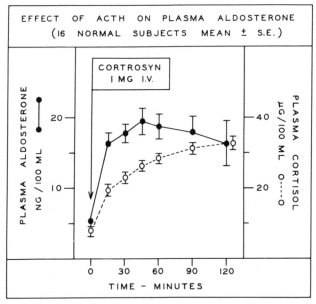

FIG. 8. Effect of intravenous Cortrosyn® on the plasma levels of aldosterone and cortisol in 16 normal subjects. *Each point and vertical bar,* mean ± SE. (From Kowarski et al., ref. 1.)

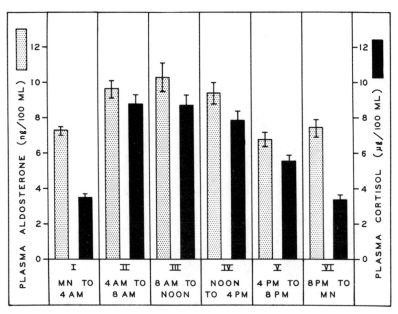

FIG. 9. Mean 4-hr integrated concentration of plasma aldosterone levels in eight normal subjects. (From Kowarski et al., ref. 1.)

compared to values obtained from normal, nonpregnant adults in supine positions on similar dietary conditions. Cord plasma aldosterone concentrations were slightly, but significantly, higher than those of the corresponding mothers (1). It is of great interest to note that the levels of infants born to mothers on low-sodium diet and/or diuretics were markedly higher than those of infants born to mothers on normal sodium diet. Furthermore, the levels remained elevated at 72 hr of life. It is not known how fast the levels returned to normal, nor is the mechanism for the elevated concentrations understood at this time.

These findings indicate that normal newborn infants require higher aldosterone concentrations than adults and are able to further increase their levels in response to sodium depletion in their mothers. Low-sodium diet in normal infants and children (7) will also result in an increase in aldosterone secretion rate as shown in Fig. 11.

SUMMARY

In summary, we have shown that:

(a) The fetus produces a large portion of its aldosterone, and its plasma levels are higher than those of the mothers.

(b) At birth, the plasma levels are similar to those of erect adults, but higher than supine adults.

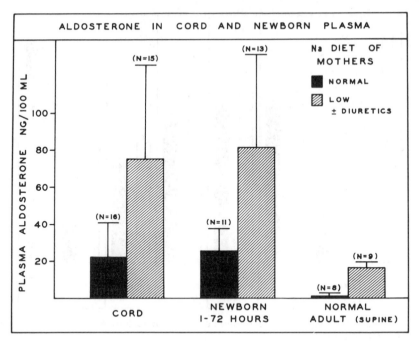

FIG. 10. Aldosterone concentration in cord and newborn plasma. These values are compared to values obtained on normal, nonpregnant adults in a supine position on similar dietary conditions. *Dark bars,* mothers receiving normal sodium intake; *shaded bars,* sodium-depleted mothers. (From Beitins et al., ref. 11.)

(c) The aldosterone secretion rate during the first week of life is about one-third that found later in life, which remains unchanged despite the increase in body size.

(d) The MCR of aldosterone probably does not change much at various ages when corrected for body size. Hence, the higher plasma levels of aldosterone during the first year of life are related to the higher secretion rate in relation to body size.

(e) Both fetus and child can respond to sodium depletion by an increase in their plasma aldosterone concentration.

ACKNOWLEDGMENTS

This work was supported by Research Grants R01-HD-06284-04, AM-00180-22, Traineeship Grant T1-AM-5219, and Research Career Award 5K06-AM-21855-12 (CJM) of the National Institutes of Health, United States Public Health Service.

The patients were studied in the Clinical Research Center of Pediatrics, supported by Grant 5-M01-RR-3352 from the General Clinical Research Cen-

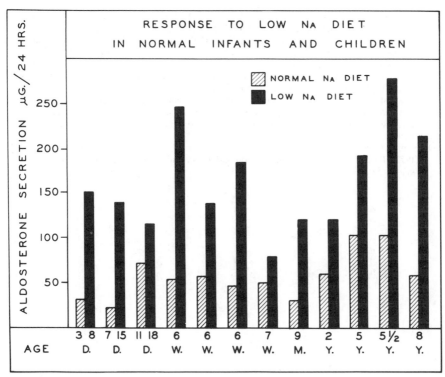

FIG. 11. Response of aldosterone secretion rate of 12 infants and children to low-sodium diet. (From Weldon et al., ref. 7.)

ters Program of the Division of Research Resources, National Institutes of Health.

REFERENCES

1. Kowarski, A., de Lacerda, L., and Migeon, C. J. (1975): Integrated concentration of plasma aldosterone in normal subjects: Correlation with cortisol. *J. Clin. Endocrinol. Metab.,* 40:204–210.
2. Nowaczynski, W., Kuchel, O., and Genest, J. (1971): A decreased metabolic clearance rate of aldosterone in benign essential hypertension. *J. Clin. Invest.,* 50:2184–2190.
3. Genest, J., Nowaczynski, W., Kuchel, C., Henerli, R., Boucher, R., and Rojo-Ortega, M. (1975): Mineralocorticoid activity in patients in the early benign phase of essential hypertension. *J. Steroid Biochem.,* 6:755–760.
4. Migeon, C. J. (1965): Adrenal cortex-visualizing disorders. In: *The Diagnosis and Treatment of Endocrine Disorders in Childhood and Adolescence,* edited by L. Wilkins, pp. 418–419. Charles C Thomas, Springfield, Ill.
5. Kenny, F. M., Malvaux, P., and Migeon, C. J. (1963): Cortisol production rate in newborns, infants and children. *Pediatrics,* 31:360–373.
6. Migeon, C. J., Green, O. C., and Eckert, J. P. (1963): Study of adrenocortical function in obesity. *Metabolism,* 12:718–739.

7. Weldon, V. V., Kowarski, A., and Migeon, C. J. (1967): Aldosterone secretion rates in normal subjects from infancy to adulthood. *Pediatrics,* 39:713–723.
8. Kowarski, A., Katz, H., and Migeon, C. J. (1974): Plasma aldosterone concentration in normal subjects from infancy to adulthood. *J. Clin. Endocrinol. Metab.* 38:489–491.
9. Kowarski, A., Finkelstein, J. W., Spaulding, J. S., Holman, G. H., and Migeon, C. J. (1965): Aldosterone secretion rate in congenital adrenal hyperplasia: A discussion of the theories on the pathogenesis of the salt-losing form of the syndrome. *J. Clin. Invest.,* 44:1505–1513.
10. Kowarski, A. A. (1976): On the mechanism of salt-loss in congenital adrenal hyperplasia. In: *International Symposium on the Treatment of Congenital Adrenal Hyperplasia,* edited by C. J. Migeon, A. A. Kowarski, L. Plotnick, and P. Lee. University Park Press, Baltimore, Md., *in press.*
11. Beitins, I. Z., Bayard, F., Levitsky, L., Ances, I. G., Kowarski, A., and Migeon, C. J. (1972): Plasma aldosterone concentration at delivery and during the newborn period. *J. Clin. Invest.,* 51:383–394.

Juvenile Hypertension, edited by
M. I. New and L. S. Levine. Raven
Press, New York © 1977.

Familial, Dexamethasone-Suppressible, Normokalemic Hyperaldosteronism

C. E. Grim, M. H. Weinberger, and S. K. Anand

Department of Medicine, Specialized Center of Research in Hypertension, Indiana University School of Medicine, Indianapolis, Indiana 46202

INTRODUCTION

The syndrome of dexamethasone-suppressible hyperaldosteronism has been observed in four separate individuals (1–4). Investigation of other family members revealed additional cases in three of the four families (1,2,4). The index cases in all of these previous reports were identified by the presence of moderate to severe hypertension and spontaneous hypokalemia. Further investigations detected suppressed plasma renin activity and increased urinary aldosterone excretion. The administration of dexamethasone returned blood pressure to normal and the biochemical evidence of hyperaldosteronism disappeared. During the last 2 years (5), we have been investigating a family (father and two boys ages 8 and 6) with a similar, but less severe, syndrome that is also dexamethasone suppressible. A unique feature of this family is that hypokalemia was not observed consistently. Initially, suspicion of mineralo-corticoid hypertension was aroused by the finding of very low renin levels obtained as a routine portion of a work-up for the etiology of the hypertension. Without the measurement of renin levels, these children and their father would have been said to have essential hypertension.

Case Report

The proband, an 8-year-old boy (son 1), was found to have elevated blood pressure of 140/88 mm Hg on a routine physical examination for grade school athletics. Hypertension had been discovered in the 31-year-old father, of Dutch–Indonesian extraction, 3 years earlier, and he had been evaluated for secondary hypertension by his family physician 2 years previously. The father's serum electrolytes, renal function, and renal arteriogram were normal; renin levels were not measured. The diagnosis of essential hypertension was made and his blood pressure responded to diuretics and α-methyldopa (Aldomet®); however, he stopped taking medication when he felt well. Because of the elevated blood pressure in son 1, the family physician obtained an electrocardiogram that was compatible with left ventricular hypertrophy. When the proband's younger brother (son 2) was examined, his blood pressure was also found to be elevated. Both children were then referred to the Riley Children's Hospital for further evaluation.[1]

The two children were the products of full-term normal pregnancies. Early growth and development had been normal. Although neither child had a history of serious illness, both had experienced occasional nose bleeds since approximately 5 years of age. On physical examination, blood pressure was elevated at 144/88 in the younger boy and 140/90 in the older boy. The initial physical examination was otherwise normal in both children and no abdominal bruits could be heard. The initial laboratory evaluation revealed that the serum electrolytes were normal as was an SMA-12 and urinalysis. Creatinine clearance, urinary excretion of 17-hydroxy- and ketosteroids, and diurnal measurements of plasma cortisol were normal. This initial evaluation in the hospital revealed no evidence for a secondary form of hypertension. In view of the history of hypertension in the father and his family, it was felt that both boys and the father probably had essential hypertension. However, during this first hospitalization, a recumbent overnight peripheral plasma renin activity was 0.1 ng angiotensin I/ml/3 hr in both children; this is much below our normal adult values. The father and two sons were subsequently hospitalized in the Indiana University Clinical Research Center for further investigation. Genotyping was compatible with paternity.

METHODS

Plasma renin activity (PRA) (6) and plasma aldosterone (PA) (7) were performed by techniques previously reported. Plasma cortisol (PC) was performed by specific radioimmunoassay (8). Serum electrolytes were performed by flame photometry. Urinary aldosterone (UA) excretion was determined by the New England Nuclear Company, Boston, Massachusetts.

Study Period No. 1 (November 1973)

The purpose of this investigation was to observe the dynamic response of PRA, PA, and UA excretion to high-sodium intake, low-sodium intake, and to saline infusion (9). The subjects were placed on a constant diet containing 2 meq sodium/kg body weight. The potassium intake was also constant at 70 meq potassium/day for the father and 60 meq potassium/day for the children.

---
[1]We should like to thank Drs. Robert Armer and Paul Williams for referring these patients to us for evaluation.

After 3 days on the constant diet, the diurnal variation of PRA, PA, and PC was determined from 8 a.m. to 8 p.m. by measuring these variables every 4 hr. The 8-a.m. sample was obtained after overnight recumbency and when the subjects arose and remained standing or walking 50 min/hr until 8 p.m. (10). On the sixth day, a saline infusion was given. On the ninth day, sodium intake was decreased to 10 meq/day. The low-sodium diet samples were obtained on the twelfth day.

Response to Saline Infusion and Low-Sodium Diet

As can be seen in Fig. 1, the 2-hr upright peripheral PRA before a saline infusion was below our lower limit of normal. PA, obtained at the same time, was within our normal range. The subjects then assumed the recumbent position for intravenous saline administration. The children and their father received 1 and 2 liters of saline, respectively, over the next 4 hr. At the end of this infusion (noon), PRA, shown in the middle portion of Fig. 1, was at or below the lower limit of our normal adult range in all three subjects. However, as shown in the upper portion of the figure, PA failed to suppress into the normal adult range in any of the subjects. The right portion of Fig. 1 demonstrates the results of PRA and PA after 2 hr of upright posture when the patients had achieved sodium balance on a 10 meq sodium diet for 4 days. Peripheral PRA was still markedly below normal. PA levels, shown on a different scale than to the left of Fig. 1, did not change with the low-sodium diet. These results demonstrated that PA did not suppress normally with saline infusion or increase normally with sodium depletion; this, coupled with the marked suppression of PRA, suggested autonomy of aldosterone production.

Urinary Steroid Analysis

Table 1 shows the excretion rates of some urinary steroids. In the father, aldosterone excretion was normal ($< 22 \mu g/24$ hr) on 2 of the 3 days on a high-sodium intake. The two sons were probably in the high-normal range for children. Tetrahydroaldosterone (TH-ALDO), 18-hydroxytetrahydrodeoxy-corticosterone (18-OH-TH-DOC), and deoxycorticosterone (DOC) excretions[2] were in the normal adult range. The excretion of 17-hydroxy- and 17-ketosteroids was normal.

Circadian Rhythm

Figure 2 depicts the changes in PRA, PA, and PC during a high-sodium intake over a 12-hr period in the father and two sons. As can be seen in this

---

[2]Kindly determined by Dr. James Melby, Boston, Massachusetts.

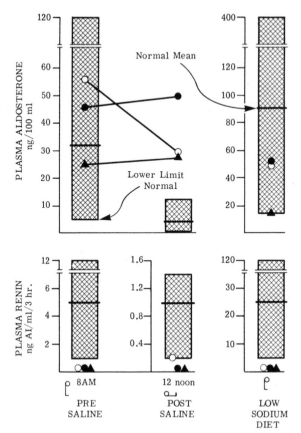

FIG. 1. Study period no. 1. PRA and PA in the father (▲), son 1 (●), and son 2 (○). The presaline sample was obtained at 8 a.m. after 2 hr of upright posture. The postsaline sample was obtained at noon at the end of a 4-hr saline infusion, while the subjects were recumbent. The subjects were ingesting a 2 meq/kg body weight dietary sodium intake. The low-sodium diet samples were obtained at 8 a.m. (2 hr upright) after 4 days on a 10 meq sodium intake. *Shaded bars,* normal adult ranges; *horizontal bars,* normal adult mean.

illustration, base-line PRA was extremely low throughout the day; PA levels in recumbency were elevated. With 2 hr of upright posture, two of the three subjects had elevated peripheral PA levels. However, at noon, with continued upright posture, PA was in the normal range and was generally normal at other times of the day. PC, shown in the upper portion of Fig. 2, followed a normal pattern, with the highest values at 8 a.m. and the lowest at 8 p.m.

Study Period No. 2 (January to February 1974)

Because of the demonstration of suppressed PRA, failure of PA to suppress normally with saline infusion and the normal to elevated UA excretion, as well

TABLE 1. Excretion rates of urinary steroids

Steroid	Father				Son 1				Son 2			
	D3	D4	D5	D11	D3	D4	D5	D11	D3	D4	D5	D11
UA excretion[a]	17.4	13.9	31.1	14	10.6	10.5	13.3	6	13.3	12.5	11.9	8
Sodium excretion[b]	215	150	217	35	60	56	61	12	53	53	65	18
TH-ALDO[a]	49	25				33	23			55	15	
18-OH-TH-DOC[a]	41	14				14	13			26	30	
DOC[a]		26					5			14	15	
17-Hydroxysteroids[c]	6.3					3.5				2.9		
17-Ketosteroids[c]	9.4					1.5				1.4		

[a] μg/24 hr.
[b] meq/24 hr.
[c] mg/24 hr.

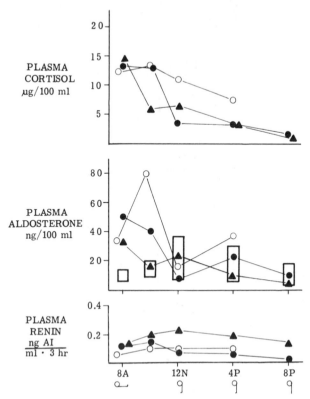

FIG. 2. Postural and diurnal changes over a 12-hr period. Posture is indicated at the bottom of the figure : ᴑ recumbent, ᑫ standing.

as the apparent familial nature of the disturbance, we considered the possibility that this family represented a mild variant of the syndrome(s) described by several investigators; hypertension, hypokalemia, low PRA, and elevated aldosterone secretion and excretion reversed by the administration of dexamethasone. Therefore, an outpatient investigation of the effects of dexamethasone on blood pressure, PRA, PC, PA, UA and 17-hydroxysteroid excretion, and serum potassium was undertaken. The father and the sons received 0.5 and 0.25 mg of dexamethasone, respectively, every 6 hr (Fig. 3).

Blood Pressure Responses

Both children had a rapid decrease in blood pressure between the first and second week of dexamethasone administration. However, the blood pressure in the father did not decrease to normal levels until after the second week of treatment. With the cessation of dexamethasone therapy, hypertension returned rapidly in the father. However, the children required over 1 month to reach frankly hypertensive levels again.

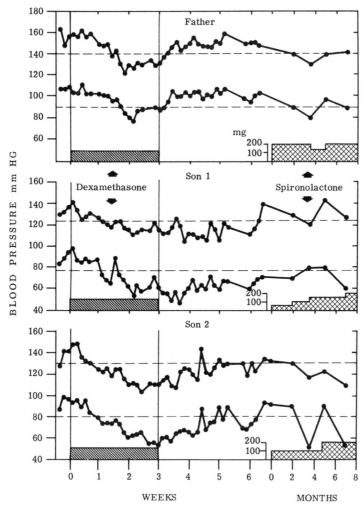

FIG. 3 Study period no. 2. Changes in blood pressure with dexamethasone *(left)* and spironolactone *(right)*.

Biochemical Response

Figure 4 depicts biochemical changes with dexamethasone administration. PRA rose from a median value of 0.2 ng angiotensin I/ml/hr at the control period to a median value of 1 ng angiotensin I/ml/hr after 2 weeks of treatment. Two weeks after the cessation of dexamethasone, peripheral PRA had decreased to control levels (week 5). PC decreased during dexamethasone administration and returned to normal levels following cessation. Although not shown, urinary 17-hydroxy- and ketosteroids decreased to barely detectable levels with dexamethasone and returned to control values afterward. The

CHANGES WITH DEXAMETHASONE

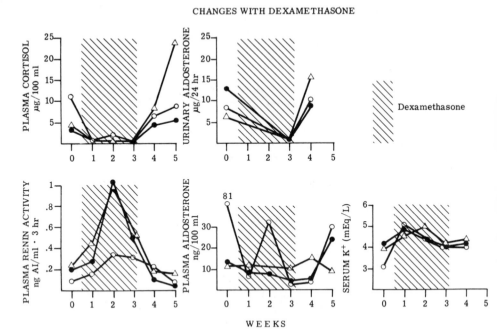

FIG. 4. Study period no. 2. Changes in biochemical parameters with dexamethasone therapy. Subjects indicated as in Fig. 1 (see text).

middle portion of Fig. 4 depicts the response of PA and UA excretion. It can be seen that at the end of 3 weeks of therapy, PA was decreased from control observations and UA excretion had decreased to essentially undetectable levels. One week after the cessation of dexamethasone, UA excretion levels had returned to normal; however, changes in PA were not as consistent. The right-hand portion of Fig. 4 depicts the changes in serum potassium. There was a tendency for serum potassium to increase with dexamethasone administration. It should be emphasized that we rarely found serum potassium levels less than 3.6 in either the father or the two children.

A trial of therapy with spironolactone was undertaken and the results are shown in Fig. 3. The father achieved normotension with this drug at a dose of 200 mg/day. However, with long-term therapy, he developed bilateral painful gynecomastia and spironolactone was discontinued. Both children were controlled with spironolactone but they also required 200 mg/day.

Study Period No. 3 (August 1975)

To further investigate the time course of these changes, the subjects were rehospitalized in August 1975 for further balance studies. All drugs had been discontinued for 2 months before admission. The protocol that was followed during this hospitalization was as follows: two days prior to hospital admission (days 1 and 2 in Fig. 5), the subjects collected daily 24-hr urine samples. They were admitted to the hospital on day 3 and ingested a constant diet during the rest of the hospitalization. Sodium intake was fixed at 2 meq/kg body weight; the father received 70 meq potassium/day and children received 60 meq/day. Blood pressure was measured four times a day and averaged. Daily 24-hr urine samples were collected for aldosterone excretion. Upright peripheral PRA, PA, and PC were obtained as indicated in Fig. 5. Dexamethasone was begun at 2 p.m. on day 6. The father and the children received 0.5 and 0.25 mg, respectively, every 6 hr.

Sodium Balance

During the first few days of study, the father appeared to be in negative sodium balance. With the administration of dexamethasone (beginning on day 6), evidence of negative sodium balance could not be demonstrated. Son 1 appeared to be eating considerable amounts of sodium as an outpatient; indeed, he was excreting more sodium than his father. Unfortunately, he was not clearly in sodium balance at the initiation of dexamethasone therapy. Nonetheless, during the therapy, urinary sodium excretion was always greater than intake. Son 2 similarly excreted considerable sodium as an outpatient and was not in apparent sodium balance at the time of initiation of dexamethasone therapy. During the treatment, his sodium excretion was always greater than his intake. Potassium balance was not significantly altered and is not shown.

Blood Pressure Response to Dexamethasone Therapy

The day following administration of dexamethasone therapy, blood pressure had decreased significantly in the father and remained lower during the hospitalization, although he never achieved diastolic pressure less than 90 mm Hg. Within 36 hr of initiation of the therapy, son 1 was normotensive and remained as such during dexamethasone administration; son 2 behaved in a similar fashion.

UA Excretion

In the father, control UA excretion averaged 6 μg/24 hr for the 3 days preceding dexamethasone administration. With the administration of dexamethasone, this rapidly decreased to less than 1 μg/24 hr. In son 1, aldosterone excretion averaged 8 μg/24 hr for 3 days prior to dexamethasone. After 36 hr of treatment, this decreased to approximately 1 μg/24 hr. Son 2, whose

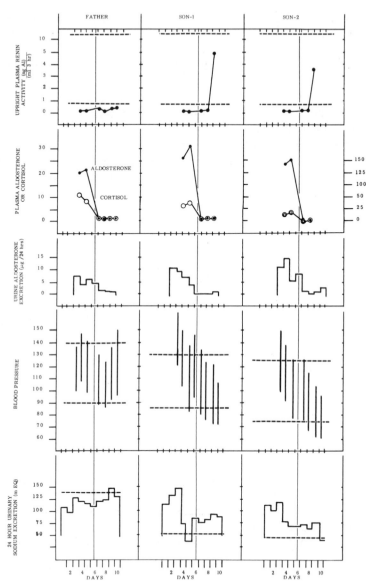

FIG. 5. Study period no. 3. Acute time course of changes with dexamethasone. The horizontal, dashed lines in the sodium excretion portion indicate the intake in each subject. The horizontal, dashed lines in the blood pressure portion indicate the normal limits (90%) for the systolic and diastolic pressure. In the PA portion of the figure, PA is expressed in ng/100 ml, PC as μg/100 ml. Note that the scale on the right-hand side for aldosterone and cortisol applies only to son 2. In the PRA section, the horizontal, dashed lines represent the normal ranges for adults in our laboratory.

urinary aldosterone excretion averaged 9 μg/24 hr prior to 3 days of dexamethasone administration, had a similar response. Within 24 hr after initiation of dexamethasone, UA excretion had decreased to 2 μg/24 hr.

Response of PA and PC to Dexamethasone Administration

In the upper portion of Fig. 5, 2-hr upright (8 a.m.) PC and PA obtained before the administration of dexamethasone was normal in the father and son 1. However, the peripheral PA level in son 2 was significantly greater than normal on the two occasions. The morning after the initiation of this therapy, PA and PC had decreased to extremely low levels and remained as such while dexamethasone was administered.

Peripheral PRA

The upper portion of Fig. 5 depicts changes in PRA (2 hr upright, 8 a.m.). Prior to dexamethasone administration, this was extremely low in all three subjects and remained as such during the initial phase of dexamethasone therapy. The father's level did not change. However, on the final day of therapy, peripheral PRA in the two sons had increased into our normal adult range.

Following discharge from the hospital, therapy for the two children was changed to prednisone (2.5 mg/day); both children have remained normotensive. The father, however, required increases up to 7.5 mg/day of prednisone to normalize the blood pressure. Peripheral PA has remained in the normal range under these conditions and peripheral PRA has increased somewhat, although not consistently into the normal adult range.

Additional Studies in the Father

Adrenal venography was attempted but no adrenal veins could be located. Adrenal iodocholesterol scan showed bilateral uptake (11). A graded infusion of ACTH was performed as previously reported (12); the results are shown in Fig. 6. There appears to be an abnormally rapid increase in PA in response to ACTH. Furthermore, at infusion rates of 50, 100, and 200 mIU/30 min, the PA was outside our normal range.

DISCUSSION

The family studied represents the fourth report of familial, glucocorticoid-suppressible primary aldosteronism (1–4,13). Without the measurement of peripheral plasma renin levels, this family was thought to have essential hypertension. The finding of suppressed PRA in the absence of overt biochemical hyperaldosteronism is present in approximately 25% of adults with

RESPONSE OF PLASMA ALDOSTERONE to ACTH$_{\alpha I-24}$ INFUSION

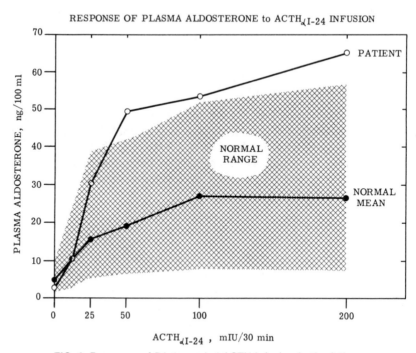

FIG. 6. Response of PA to graded ACTH infusion in the father.

"essential" hypertension (14). The incidence of such low-renin levels in children with hypertension is not known, although low-renin "essential" hypertension has been reported in children (15). The present and previously reported cases of dexamethasone-suppressible low-renin states would make it prudent to give all children and adults with low-renin "essential" hypertension a trial of dexamethasone therapy. The current report, as well as that of New and Levine (reported elsewhere in this volume), suggests that the measurement of PA or UA excretion after 2 days of dexamethasone treatment permits identification of such patients; this is attributable to the decrease in UA to undetectable levels in the three subjects, within 48 hr of initiation of therapy. The blood pressure response may take longer to determine, especially in the older subjects who have had hypertension for a longer period of time.

Dexamethasone-suppressible hypertension, with biochemical evidence of hyperaldosteronism and low-renin levels, has been reported by three other groups. The first report by Sutherland et al. (1) of a father and son with suppressed plasma renin and obvious hyperaldosteronism differed from the present one in that there were intermittent elevations in 17-keto- and 17-hydroxysteroids. The case reported by New and Peterson (2,13) likewise presented with overt biochemical evidence of hyperaldosteronism. A rapid decrease in aldosterone excretion with dexamethasone was documented. Miura et al. (3) reported a 17-year-old girl with similar findings but low-normal 17-hydroxysteroid excretion. The family reported by Giebink et al. (4) differed from the present and other reported cases in that there was considerable delay in aldosterone suppression with dexamethasone.

No consistent evidence for an adrenal steroid biosynthetic defect has been presented in the present or other reported cases. It seems clear that the aldosterone production in these cases is primarily controlled by a dexamethasone-suppressible factor rather than by the renin–angiotensin system or by serum potassium. There appear to be two other major possibilities. The first is that there is some unknown dexamethasone-suppressible, aldosterone-stimulating factor present in these patients. We chose to dismiss this possibility at the present based on the lack of evidence for such a factor in man. We suggest another hypothesis: the defect in these patients is caused by an abnormal adrenal receptor for ACTH in the aldosterone-producing adrenal cells. The abnormality of this receptor is such that when it reacts with normal levels of ACTH, it causes greater than normal production of aldosterone from these cells. This appears to be supported by the increased response of PA to graded ACTH infusion seen in the father. Careful dose–response curves in these patients should be instructive.

The important message for the clinician and epidemiologist is that hypertension in childhood, as in adults, can no longer be assumed to be "essential" even in the presence of normal physical examination, normal intravenous pyelography, normal serum electrolytes, and normal UA excretion. Careful renin measurements in hypertensive children will undoubtedly reveal more cases of dexamethasone-suppressible hypertension.

ACKNOWLEDGMENTS

This work was supported in part by grants HL 1459, Specialized Center of Research (SCOR) in Hypertension; RR 00750, Clinical Research Center; and HL 20034, Hypertension: Psychophysiologic and Genetic Precursors.

Portions of these studies were presented at the 47th Annual Meeting of the Central Society for Clinical Research, Chicago, Illinois, November 1974.

REFERENCES

1. Sutherland, D. J. A., Ruse, R. L., and Laidlaw, J. C. (1966): Hypertension, increased aldosterone secretion and low plasma renin activity relieved by dexamethasone. *Can. Med. Assoc. J.,* 95:1109–1119.
2. New, M. I., and Peterson, R. E. (1967): A new form of congenital adrenal hyperplasia. *J. Clin. Endocrinol. Metab.,* 27:300–305.

3. Miura, K., Yoshinaga, K., Goto, K., Katsushima, I., Maebashi, M., Demura, H., Iino, M., Demura, R., and Torikai, T. (1968): A case of glucocorticoid-responsive hyperaldosteronism. *J. Clin. Endocrinol. Metab.*, 28:1807–1815.
4. Giebink, G. S., Gotlin, R. W., Biglieri, E. G., and Katz, F. A. (1973): A kindred with familial glucocorticoid-suppressible aldosteronism. *J. Clin. Endocrinol Metab.*, 36:715–723.
5. Grim, C. E., Weinberger, M. H., Anand, S. K., and Northway, J. D. (1974): Familial, normokalemic, glucocorticoid-suppressible hyperaldosteronism. *Clin. Res.*, 22:632A.
6. Weinberger, M. H., Ramsdell, J. W., Rosner, D. R., and Geddes, J. J. L. (1972): Effect of chlorothiazide and sodium on vascular responsiveness to angiotensin II. *Am. J. Physiol.*, 223:1049–1052.
7. Gomez-Sanchez, C., Kem, D. C., and Kaplan, N. M. (1973): A radioimmunoassay for plasma aldosterone by immunologic purification. *J. Clin. Endocrinol. Metab.*, 36:795–798.
8. Gomez-Sanchez, C., Holland, O. B., and Milewich, L. (1976): Radioiodinated derivatives of steroids for radioimmunoassay: Application to the radioimmunoassay of cortisol. *J. Clin. Endocrinol. Metab., submitted for publication.*
9. Kem, D. C., Weinberger, M. H., Mayes, D., and Nugent, C. A. (1971): Saline suppression of plasma aldosterone in hypertension. *Arch. Intern. Med.*, 128:380–386.
10. Grim, C. E., and Keitzer, W. F. (1974): Circadian rhythm in unilateral renovascular hypertension. *Ann. Intern. Med.*, 80:298–304.
11. Conn, J. W., Beierwaltes, W. H., Lieberman, L. M., Ansari, A. N., Cohen, E. L., Bookstein, J. J., and Herwig, K. R. (1971): Primary aldosteronism: Preoperative tumor visualization by scintillation scanning. *J. Clin. Endocrinol. Metab.*, 33:713–716.
12. Kem, D. D., Gomez-Sanchez, C., Kramer, N. J., Holland, D. B., and Higgins, J. T. (1975): Plasma aldosterone and renin activity response to ACTH infusion in dexamethasone-suppressed normal and sodium-depleted man. *J. Clin. Endocrinol. Metab.*, 40:116–124.
13. New, M. I., Siegel, E. J., and Peterson, R. E. (1973): Dexamethasone-suppressible hyperaldosteronism. *J. Clin. Endocrinol. Metab.*, 37:93–100.
14. Kaplan, N. M. (1973): *Clinical Hypertension.* Medcom Press, New York.
15. Gruskin, A. B., Linshaw, M., Cote, M. L., and Fleisher, D. S. (1971): Low-renin essential hypertension—Another form of childhood hypertension. *J. Pediatr.*, 78:765–771.

Juvenile Hypertension, edited by
M. I. New and L. S. Levine. Raven
Press, New York © 1977.

A Syndrome of Low-Renin Hypertension in Children

*Jeremy S. D. Winter and John K. McKenzie

*Department of Pediatrics, Endocrinology Section, Health Sciences Centre,
University of Manitoba, Winnipeg, Manitoba R3E OW1; and Department of
Medicine, Nephrology Section, Health Sciences Centre, University of Manitoba,
Winnipeg, Manitoba R3E OZ3, Canada*

A primary disorder of excessive mineralocorticoid secretion should be suspected when a patient presents with the following problems: (a) arterial hypertension; (b) hypokalemia and alkalosis secondary to urinary potassium wasting; and (c) suppressed plasma renin activity. Further support for the diagnosis arises if these features can be corrected by a mineralocorticoid antagonist such as spironolactone, but final confirmation requires documentation of excessive or inappropriate secretion of a potent mineralocorticoid such as aldosterone or desoxycorticosterone.

Mineralocorticoid excess is often equated with aldosterone excess. Aldosterone-secreting adrenal adenomas as a cause of primary aldosteronism are rare in children (16); aldosterone excess is more commonly associated with the syndromes of bilateral nodular adrenal hyperplasia (2) or glucocorticoid-responsive hyperaldosteronism (10). But hypertension can also result from excessive secretion of other mineralocorticoids such as corticosterone or desoxycorticosterone, which occur in association with congenital deficiencies of adrenal 11β- or 17α-hydroxylase (4).

It is the purpose of this report to describe two unrelated children who show clinical features strongly suggestive of inappropriate mineralocorticoid secretion. Both have low-renin hypertension and metabolic alkalosis that can be corrected by spironolactone. However, to date, we have not been able to demonstrate excessive secretion of any known mineralocorticoid.

CASE REPORTS

Patient L. C. This boy, of mixed European-American Indian descent, was first seen at age 19 months because of increasing projectile vomiting, polyuria, and polydipsia since age 3 months. His height growth was adequate (10th percentile), but he was malnourished and moderately dehydrated. His blood pressure was 140/100. Urine pH was 6.0 and specific gravity 1.005. Blood urea nitrogen was 18 mg/dl. Serum electrolyte concentrations are shown in Table 1. A clinical diagnosis of pyloric stenosis was confirmed by X-rays. He underwent a modified Ramstedt pyloromyotomy, and the vomiting ceased.

When seen a few weeks later, his blood pressure ranged from 90/55 to 145/90, and he was still hypokalemic and alkalotic. He had been on a normal diet and was no longer vomiting. Stool electrolyte losses were negligible (Na^+ 0.3 to 0.7 meq/day; K^+ 1.8 to 2.0 meq/day; Cl^- 0.4 to 0.7 meq/day). Sweat chloride concentration was 19.4 meq/liter.

In spite of his hypokalemia, his urinary potassium ranged from 20 to 50 meq/day. With a markedly restricted sodium intake (10 meq/day) and supplementary potassium, he was able to raise his serum potassium as high as 3.5 meq/liter. But on a high-sodium intake (100 meq/day), his serum potassium fell to 1.5 meq/liter.

Meanwhile, several causes of hypertension and hypokalemia were excluded. He showed normal blood pressure responses to phentolamine and histamine, and his urinary vanillylmandelic acid (VMA) was 0.85 mg/24 hr. No 5-hydroxyindole-acetic acid was detected in his urine. During a graded angiotensin infusion (from 4.5 up to 18.1 ng/kg/min), his blood pressure rose to 195/150. Urinary steroid excretion was normal: 17-ketosteroid (17-KS) 0.5 mg/24 hr; 17-hydroxycorticos-teroid (17-OH-CS) 0.3 mg/24 hr; pregnanediol and pregnanetriol both less than 0.05 mg/24 hr. His serum cortisol concentration was 17.1 μg/dl at 8 a.m. and 10.6 μg/dl at 3 p.m.

After several weeks of potassium repletion, his endogenous creatinine clear-ance was 95 ml/min/1.73 m^2 and his maximum urine specific gravity after pitressin was 1.015; there was no aminoaciduria or glycosuria. During ammonium chloride loading, his urine pH fell to 5.0; the urine was free of bicarbonate and showed a normal rise in titratable acidity and ammonia excretion. Intravenous and retro-grade pyelography showed mild dilatation of the right calyces, pelvis, and proxi-mal two-thirds of the ureter; a voiding cystourethrogram was normal. A closed renal biopsy showed six normal glomeruli, with normal small vessels and convo-luted tubules. No juxtaglomerular apparatus was identified. Beginning abruptly at the corticomedullary junction, the architecture of the pyramid was distorted by prominent interstitial fibrosis and large areas of nephrocalcinosis. The calcium

TABLE 1. *Electrolyte concentrations*

Age	Remarks	Blood pH	Serum			
			Na⁺	K⁺	Cl⁻	HCO₃⁻
Patient L. C.						
1 yr 7 mo	Pyloric stenosis	—	153	3.1	105	26.4
1 yr 9 mo	No therapy	7.40–7.54	148–155	1.5–2.5	105–115	22.3–36.4
	Spironolactone		138–145	4.4–5.5		
2–4 yr	Triamterene	7.34–7.43	132–156	4.2–5.5	102–116	20.2–24.7
4–5 yr	Triamterene	7.41–7.50	141–145	3.1–4.1	108–113	24.0–27.0
5 yr 9 mo	Nil	7.46	150	2.2	107	32.0
5 yr 10 mo–9 yr	Spironolactone	7.38–7.45	131–147	4.2–5.5	105–109	20.0–25.0
Patient M. T.						
3 wk	Pyloric stenosis	7.69	141	3.2	79	31.4
	Postsurgery	7.49	143	2.5–3.7	102–108	33.5
2 yr 9 mo	No therapy	7.45	148	2.5–2.8	102	31.7
3–6 yr	Spironolactone	7.31–7.43	134–149	3.8–5.3	106–112	17.5–23.5

was deposited in the walls of the loops of Henle and distal collecting tubules, primarily between the lining epithelium and the basement membrane.

Investigations of his mineralocorticoid function are shown in Table 2. The consistent suppression of plasma renin activity (normal range 1 to 5 ng/ml/hr) and his response to spironolactone initially suggested a primary disorder of excessive adrenal mineralocorticoid secretion, but surprisingly his urinary excretion rates of aldosterone and desoxycorticosterone were not elevated (normal range 4 to 20 μg/ 24 hr). After several months of therapy with potassium gluconate and spironolactone, during which time his blood pressure and serum electrolytes were normal, his aldosterone secretion rate was 24.1 μg/24 hr (normal 50 to 250 μg/24 hr). When therapy was discontinued, his hypertension and hypokalemia recurred.

At age 2 years 3 months, therapy was restarted, using the potassium-retaining diuretic triamterene (150 mg/day). Again his serum electrolytes and blood pressure became normal, and his plasma renin activity rose to 2.2 ng/ml/hr. He received triamterene for 3 years, and during this time he grew and developed normally.

By age 5 years 9 months, there was evidence of recurring hypertension, polyuria, and hypokalemia, and the triamterene was discontinued. Off therapy, his blood pressure rose as high as 190/120, but plasma renin activity and serum aldosterone levels were undetectable, even after 4 days of furosemide administration (Table 2). At this time, his renal function was normal with the exception of impaired concentrating capacity. Intravenous pyelography showed persistent mild dilatation of the right collecting system, and he underwent surgery to remove an adynamic segment of the right ureter. Both adrenals were visualized and appeared normal. Open biopsies of both kidneys showed sclerosis of several glomeruli, pericapsular and interstitial fibrosis, and small foci of calcification in the distal tubules. Juxtaglomerular hyperplasia was not observed.

Therapy was reinstituted with increasing doses of spironolactone. With 300 mg/ day, his blood pressure and serum electrolytes returned to normal. He has been on this therapy for the past 3 years and continues to grow and develop normally.

Patient M. T. This American Indian girl presented at age 3 weeks with projectile vomiting and dehydration. Urine specific gravity was 1.001 in spite of her dehydration. Serum electrolyte concentrations are shown in Table 1. A clinical diagno-

TABLE 2. *Mineralocorticoid function*

Age	Therapy	Plasma renin activity (ng/ ml/hr)	Serum		24-Hr urine	
			Aldosterone (ng/dl)	DOC[a] (ng/dl)	Aldosterone (μg)	DOC (μg)
Patient L. C.						
1 yr 9 mo	Nil	0	—	—	0.7	0.1
	Low-Na$^+$ diet	0	—	—	1.5	0.1
2 yr 3 mo	Spironolactone	0.5	—	—	—	—
	Triamterene	2.2	—	—	—	—
5 yr 3 mo	Triamterene	0.3	3.6	—	—	—
5 yr 9 mo	Nil	0	0	—	—	—
	Furosemide	0	0	—	—	—
	Spironolactone	0–0.4	47.6	—	—	—
6 yr 8 mo	Spironolactone	0.8	3.3	—	—	—
8 yr 7 mo	Spironolactone	2.2	18.7	9.2	—	—
Patient M. T.						
2 yr 9 mo	Nil	0.2	0	—	—	—
3 yr 7 mo	Spironolactone	0.2–0.4	1.2–2.3	—	—	—
5 yr 4 mo	Spironolactone		20.9	9.8	—	—

[a]DOC, deoxycorticosterone.

sis of pyloric stenosis was confirmed by X-rays. Following pyloromyotomy, her vomiting ceased but she remained hypokalemic and alkalotic.

She was not seen again until age 2 years 9 months, when she presented with acute onset of somnolence and ataxia; her blood pressure was 180/120. Neurological examination, skull X-rays, brain scan, and EEG were noncontributory. She was hypokalemic and alkalotic (Table 1), and in spite of this was excreting 50 to 90 meq of potassium in her urine each day.

Urinalysis, serum creatinine, blood urea nitrogen, intravenous pyelography, and selective renal arteriography were all normal. There was no blood pressure change with phentolamine; her VMA excretion was 0.44 mg/24 hr. Urinary 17-KS was 0.3 mg/24 hr, 17-OH-CS 2.5 mg/24 hr, and free cortisol 87 μg/24 hr.

She showed persistent suppression of plasma renin activity and serum aldosterone (Table 2) in spite of the administration of supplementary potassium and restriction of sodium (10 meq/day). Renin activity and aldosterone were also undetectable in samples obtained from each renal vein.

A trial of dexamethasone suppression was attempted, but this had to be discontinued after a few days because of hypokalemia and increasing hypertension that could not be controlled with α-methyldopa. She was then treated with increasing doses of spironolactone; a dose of 300 mg/day was effective in reducing her blood pressure to 100/60 and in correcting her hypokalemic alkalosis. She has been treated for 3 years and has grown and developed normally.

SPECIAL STUDIES

These unrelated American Indian children have a syndrome of low-renin hypertension, hypokalemia, and alkalosis, but there is no evidence of increased or inappropriate secretion of aldosterone or desoxycorticosterone. In spite of this, their abnormalities can be entirely corrected by large doses of the mineralocorticoid antagonist spironolactone. Therefore, the following studies were carried out in order to determine whether they were secreting a mineralocorticoid other than aldosterone or desoxycorticosterone.

Effects of Dietary Sodium Manipulation

On their initial evaluation, it appeared that salt restriction resulted in higher serum K^+ concentrations. Accordingly, their spironolactone was discontinued, an oral potassium supplement was provided, and the effects of a low-sodium diet (approximately 10 meq/day) and then a high-sodium diet (100 meq/day in L. C. and 50 meq/day in M. T.) were observed during sequential 5-day periods. The results (Table 3) showed that plasma renin activity was suppressed throughout and that the urinary and salivary Na^+/K^+ ratios were less than unity, as might be expected in a disorder of primary mineralocorticoid excess. A similar reversal of Na^+/K^+ ratio was seen in the sweat. Urinary sodium varied appropriately with changes in sodium intake, but urinary potassium concentrations did not change. Salt restriction did reduce total urinary potassium excretion, but only through a reduction in urine volume. Serum aldosterone levels remained undetectable.

TABLE 3. *Response to dietary NaCl manipulation*

Dose	Plasma renin (ng/ml/hr)	Serum aldosterone (ng/dl)	Serum Na$^+$ (meq/liter)	K$^+$ (meq/liter)	Urine Na$^+$ (meq/liter)	K$^+$ (meq/liter)	Saliva Na$^+$ (meq/liter)	K$^+$ (meq/liter)
Patient L. C.								
Na$^+$ 10 meq/day	0.1	0	144–151	2.6–3.5	14–26	29–54	6	41
Na$^+$ 100 meq/day	0.1	0	145–148	2.5–4.4	48–64	34–35		
Patient M. T.								
Na$^+$ 10 meq/day	0	0	144–145	4.2–5.1	8–13	63–64	4	34
Na$^+$ 50 meq/day	0	0	143–144	3.9–4.9	24–40	52–53	14	32

Bioassayable Mineralocorticoid Excretion

Dichloromethane extracts of urine from these patients were assayed for total mineralocorticoid activity (by bioassay) and aldosterone content (by radioimmunoassay) by Drs. Ronald Brown and Grant Liddle, Vanderbilt University. Their bioassay is based on the urinary Na$^+$/K$^+$ ratio of adrenalectomized rats after injection of the extract; results are expressed in terms of aldosterone equivalents (14). The results (Table 4) show a marked discrepancy; significant amounts of mineralocorticoid activity were measured by bioassay, but only negligible amounts of aldosterone were found by radioimmunoassay. At present, these studies are being extended to include analysis of the mineralocorticoid activity of these urines after specific hydrolysis of glucuronide and sulfate conjugates. It is not possible to state whether the amounts of mineralocorticoid activity detected by bioassay are sufficient to explain the syndrome.

Studies of Adrenal Steroidogenesis

Although these patients do not fit into any known syndrome associated with defective steroidogenesis, some studies were carried out to rule out some obscure form of congenital adrenal hyperplasia. Urinary 17-KS and 17-OH-CS were normal. Although aldosterone levels were suppressed, they (and also serum desoxycorticosterone levels) rose during treatment with spironolactone. There was no evidence for excessive accumulation of any steroid

TABLE 4. *Comparison of mineralocorticoid activity by bioassay and aldosterone concentration by radioimmunoassay in dichloromethane extracts of urine*

Patient	Bioassay activity (μg aldosterone eq/liter)	Aldosterone concentration (μg/liter)
L. C.	0.30	0.03
M. T.	1.21	0.02

TABLE 5. *Serum steroid concentrations during spironolactone therapy*

Steroid	L. C.	M. T.	Normal range
Pregnenolone	80	110	30–200
17-Hydroxypregnenolone	30	70	20–400
Progesterone	20	20	20–60
17-Hydroxyprogesterone	130	45	12–75
Androstenedione	12	14	7–20
Testosterone	15	12	3–15
Estradiol	< 0.5	< 0.5	< 1.0
11-Desoxycorticosterone	9.2	9.8	5–15
Aldosterone	18.7	20.9	2–14
11-Desoxycortisol	0	0	< 2.5
Cortisol	10.0	11.0	7–22

Serum concentrations expressed in nanograms/deciliter except for 11-desoxycortisol and cortisol, which are in micrograms/deciliter.

precursors (Table 5). Cortisol levels in serum and urine rose normally after ACTH, as did serum levels of other steroids measured (Table 6). The relative concentrations of Na^+ and K^+ in serum, urine, and saliva were not changed by ACTH administration, an indication that ACTH-dependent mineralocorticoid excess was unlikely.

Responses to Dexamethasone and Aminoglutethimide

The effects of short-term suppression of ACTH by dexamethasone (1 mg/day for 7 days) and of short-term inhibition of steroidogenesis by aminoglu-

TABLE 6. *Response to ACTH[a]*

Steroid	Patient L. C.		Patient M. T.	
	Basal	Post-ACTH	Basal	Post-ACTH
Serum[b]				
Cortisol	4.6	> 40	5.4	> 40
11-Desoxycortisol	0	6	0	0
17-Hydroxyprogesterone	10	90	6	150
Progesterone	< 10	50	< 10	32
Aldosterone	0.6	2.4	1.2	0
Na^+/K^+	147/3.6	147/3.2	144/4.1	143/3.2
Urine[c]				
Cortisol	33	1,200	64	693
Na^+/K^+	44/76	43/34	37/57	10/16
Salivary[d]				
Na^+/K^+	28/39	15/24	22/34	14/31

[a]Synacthen ® 0.5 mg i.m. × 4 days.
[b]Serum steroid levels in nanograms/deciliter except for cortisol and 11-desoxycortisol, which are in micrograms/deciliter.
[c]Urine steroid levels in micrograms/24 hr.
[d]Na^+ and K^+ concentrations in milliequivalents/liter.

TABLE 7. *Responses to dexamethasone[a] and aminoglutethimide[b]*

Steroid	Patient L. C.			Patient M. T.		
	Control	Dexameth.	Aminoglut.	Control	Dexameth.	Aminoglut.
Blood pressure	120/70	120/70	115/60	125/80	145/100	120/65
Serum Na$^+$/K$^+$	143/4.1	142/4.3	145/4.9	144/3.9	139/4.1	143/3.7
Urine Na$^+$/K$^+$	27/95	68/76	28/73	25/67	71/49	27/72
Saliva Na$^+$/K$^+$	17/25	22/21	31/16	6/16	41/43	15/26
Serum cortisol	4.6	2.4	—	5.4	2.4	—
Serum aldosterone	0.6	1.2	2.4	1.2	0	0
Plasma renin activity	0.3	0.2	0.2	0.2	0	0.2

[a]0.25 mg every hr for 7 days.
[b]125 mg every 6 hr for 7 days.

tethimide (500 mg/day for 7 days) were observed (Table 7). Neither regimen produced any consistent change in blood pressure, plasma renin activity, or Na$^+$/K$^+$ ratios in serum, saliva, or urine. Although the studies were of short duration, these negative results do not lend support to the hypothesis of excessive adrenal mineralocorticoid secretion. Since urinary cortisol excretion was not reduced during the aminoglutethimide study, administration of a larger dose is being planned.

DISCUSSION

We have described two children with hypokalemic alkalosis and low-renin hypertension who have been treated successfully with spironolactone. However, we have been unable to document excessive or autonomous secretion of known mineralocorticoids; they have no apparent enzymatic defect in steroidogenesis (e.g., 17α-hydroxylase deficiency) that might be expected to cause low-renin hypertension. The urinary bioassay data, similar to the clinical response to spironolactone, do however suggest the presence of an unidentified mineralocorticoid.

If this disorder is not due to mineralocorticoid excess, it may represent a defect in renal handling of sodium and potassium, such that the renal tubules are inordinately efficient at Na$^+$/K$^+$ exchange, even in the presence of minimal levels of mineralocorticoid. In many ways, these patients resemble children with pseudoaldosteronism, a familial syndrome characterized by low-renin hypertension, metabolic alkalosis, and suppressed levels of aldosterone secretion (9,11). There is evidence to suggest a generalized abnormality of sodium transport in pseudoaldosteronism (7); however, patients with pseudoaldosteronism do not respond to spironolactone, whereas in our study a response was noted.

Gruskin et al. (8) have reported on a child with low-renin hypertension who was unresponsive to glucocorticoid administration. This child had low salivary and sweat Na$^+$/K$^+$ ratios, low-normal serum potassium levels, and normal levels of aldosterone secretion; as in our patients the hypertension was corrected with spironolactone. Sann et al. (17) have recently described a 4-year-old girl with a similar syndrome of low-renin hypertension and hypokalemic alkalosis who improved after treatment with triamterene and spironolactone, but who also improved after administration of dexamethasone (4 mg/day for 21 days).

Various other forms of congenital hypokalemic alkalosis have been reported in which a defect in renal Na^+/K^+ transport has been implicated (3,6, 15). However, in these syndromes, the patients were not hypertensive, there was evidence of increased renin production, and there was no beneficial response to spironolactone.

It is of some interest to speculate about the possible relationships between the hypertrophic pyloric stenosis and the electrolyte abnormality in our patients. Certainly, chronic pyloric obstruction can cause alkalosis and hypokalemia, and in this situation the potassium deficit results, at least in part, from excessive urinary excretion of potassium (5). In turn, hypokalemia and alkalosis can result in nephrocalcinosis limited to the distal tubules, and this might be expected to cause some permanent defects in renal function (12). But such patients also show juxtaglomerular hyperplasia, because chronic potassium depletion has a stimulating effect on renin release (1,13). The suppression of plasma renin activity, together with the associated findings of low salivary and sweat Na^+/K^+ ratios, would seem to rule out the suggestion that they might have defective renal K^+ handling secondary to their pyloric stenosis. However, it is intriguing to speculate that they might have a congenital generalized disorder of Na^+/K^+ transport that is in some way responsible for their pyloric stenosis.

CONCLUSIONS

Two children with low-renin hypertension, hypokalemic alkalosis, low salivary and sweat Na^+/K^+ ratios, and suppressed aldosterone secretion are reported. In both children, the abnormalities were corrected by large amounts of spironolactone. No defect in adrenal steroidogenesis could be identified, although preliminary bioassay data suggest that they may be excreting a mineralocorticoid other than aldosterone.

As an alternative to mineralocorticoid excess, it is suggested that these children may have a congenital generalized disorder of Na^+/K^+ transport that renders their distal renal tubules inordinately responsive to small amounts of mineralocorticoid.

ACKNOWLEDGMENTS

This work was supported in part by the Medical Research Council of Canada and the Children's Hospital of Winnipeg Research Foundation. Jeremy S. D. Winter is a Queen Elizabeth II Scientist.

We would like to express gratitude for the advice provided and the assays performed for us by Drs. Ron Brown (Mayo Clinic), Grant Liddle and Ian Burr (Vanderbilt University), and Edward Biglieri (University of California), and for the assistance provided by Drs. Robert Walker and Garry Warne, Mr. Iqbal Riyaz, and Miss Emma Gulbis.

REFERENCES

1. Abbrecht, P. H., and Vander, A. J. (1970): Effects of chronic potassium deficiency on plasma renin activity. *J. Clin. Invest.,* 49:1510.
2. Baer, L., Sommers, S. C., Krakoff, L. R., Newton, M. A., and Laragh, J. H. (1970): Pseudo-primary aldosteronism: An entity distinct from true primary aldosteronism. *Circ. Res.,* 27(Suppl. I):203.
3. Bartter, F. C., Pronove, P., Gill, J. R., Jr., and MacCardle, R. C. (1962): Hyperplasia of the juxtaglomerular complex with hyperaldosteronism and hypokalemic alkalosis. *Am. J. Med.,* 33:811.
4. Biglieri, E. G., Harron, M. A., and Brust, N. (1966): 17-Hydroxylation deficiency in man. *J. Clin. Invest.,* 45:1946.
5. Burnett, C. H., Burrows, B. A., Commons, R. R., and Towery, B. T. (1950): Studies of alkalosis. II. Electrolyte abnormalities in alkalosis resulting from pyloric obstruction. *J. Clin. Invest.,* 29:175.
6. Camacho, A. M., and Blizzard, R. M. (1962): Congenital hypokalemia of probable renal origin. *Am. J. Dis. Child.,* 103:535.
7. Gardner, J. D., Lapey, A., Simopoulos, A. P., and Bravo, E. L. (1971): Abnormal membrane sodium transport in Liddle's syndrome. *J. Clin. Invest.,* 50:2253.
8. Gruskin, A. B., Linshaw, M., Cote, M. L., and Fleisher, D. S. (1971): Low-renin essential hypertension—another form of childhood hypertension. *J. Pediatr.,* 78:765.
9. Liddle, G. W., Bledsoe, T., and Coppage, W. S., Jr. (1964): A familial renal disorder simulating primary aldosteronism but with negligible aldosterone secretion. In: *Aldosterone,* edited by E. E. Baulieu and P. Robel, p. 353. Blackwell, Oxford.
10. Miura, K., Yoshinaga, K., Goto, K., Katsushima, I., Maebashi, M., Demura, H., Iino, M., Demura, R., and Torikai, T. (1968): A case of glucocorticoid-responsive hyperaldosteronism. *J. Clin. Endocrinol. Metab.,* 28:1807.
11. Ohno, F., Harada, H., Komatsu, K., Saijo, K., and Miyoshi, K. (1975): Two cases of pseudoaldosteronism (Liddle's syndrome) in siblings. *Endocrinol. Jpn.,* 22:163.
12. Pasternack, A., Perheentupa, J., Launiala, K., and Hallman, N. (1967): Kidney biopsy findings in familial chloride diarrhoea. *Acta Endocrinol. (Kbh.),* 55:1.
13. Pearson, A. J. G., Sladen, G. E., Edmonds, C. J., Tavill, A. S., Wills, M. R., and McIntyre, N. (1973): The pathophysiology of congenital chloridorrhoea. *Q. J. Med.,* 42:453.
14. Sennett, J. A., Brown, R. D., Island, D. P., Yarbro, L. R., Watson, J. T., Slaton, P. E., Hollifield, J. W., and Liddle, G. W. (1975): Evidence for a new mineralocorticoid in patients with low-renin essential hypertension. *Circ. Res.,* 36 (Suppl. I):2.
15. Walker, S. H., and Firminger, H. I. (1974): Familial renal dysplasia with sodium wasting and hypokalemic alkalosis. *Am. J. Dis. Child.,* 127:882.
16. Winter, J. S. D. (1975): Adrenal tumors in childhood. In: *Endocrine and Genetic Diseases of Childhood and Adolescence,* 2nd ed., edited by L. I. Gardner, p. 507. Saunders, Philadelphia, Pa.
17. Sann, L., Revol, A., Zachmann, M., Legrand, J. C., and Bethenod, M. (1976): Unusual low plasma renin hypertension in a child. *J. Clin. Endocrinol. Metab.,* 43:265.

Juvenile Hypertension, edited by
M. I. New and L. S. Levine. Raven
Press, New York © 1977.

A Rare but Curable Form of Hypertension: The "Page Kidney"

M. H. Weinberger, C. E. Grim, and J. P. Donohue

Departments of Medicine and Urology, Specialized Center of Research in Hypertension, Indiana University School of Medicine, Indianapolis, Indiana 46202

Page (6) first reported the experimental production of hypertension in animals by wrapping the kidney in cellophane. This procedure resulted in a dense perinephritis with subcapsular fibrosis and hypertension. Although several investigators have studied this experimental model of hypertension, the role of the renin-angiotensin system in the etiology and maintenance of hypertension is still controversial (1,4,5,7). Recently, several cases of a similar kind of perinephritis with subcapsular fibrosis have been reported in association with hypertension in humans (2,9). These cases have been primarily encountered in young males who have given a history of trauma to the flank or back area. Grim and colleagues (2) have implicated increased renal venous renin activity in blood from the involved kidney and a decrease in peripheral plasma renin activity following nephrectomy, with resultant cure of hypertension in the pathophysiology of this disorder. We should like to report our observations on two young men with severe hypertension associated with unilateral subcapsular hematomas and resultant fibrosis in whom studies strongly support a major role for the renin-angiotensin system in the pathogenesis of this unusual, but curable, form of hypertension.

MATERIALS AND METHODS

Case Reports

Patient 1. The first patient was a 19-year-old white male who was noted to have a blood pressure of 110/55 in August 1973. The patient was referred to the Indiana University Medical Center in May 1974 for evaluation of hypertension of 5 months duration. For 3 months prior to admission, the patient had noted frequent evening headaches, occasional dizziness, palpitations, and nocturia 2 to 3 times a night. He had a negative past medical history and no family history of hypertension. There

133

was no history of renal disease or flank trauma elicited from the patient. However, after surgery, his parents recalled that he had fallen from a scaffold 10 months previously and had landed on his right side.

The physical examination on admission showed a blood pressure of 160/130. The optic fundi showed arteriolar narrowing without other hypertensive changes. The abdominal examination revealed a vague fullness in the right, upper quadrant but no palpable mass and no abdominal bruits. The remainder of the physical examination was negative. Routine laboratory studies were completely normal without any abnormalities noted on examination of his urine. The endogenous creatinine clearance was 142 ml/min. Ths chest X-ray showed minimal left ventricular enlargement, and the electrocardiogram was normal.

The radiographic observations in this patient have been previously reported (8). A renal arteriogram was performed with a rapid-sequence excretory urogram. There was a delay in the appearance of the contrast material in the collecting system of the right kidney. A large avascular mass measuring 10 × 15 cm, arising outside the renal parenchyma but within the renal capsule and causing a concavity of the adjacent parenchyma, was identified. This mass caused distortion of the calyces and pelvis as well as deviation of the ureter, both anteriorally and medially. The arterial phase showed prominent alteration, splaying, and stretching of the intrarenal vessels on the right without renal arterial narrowing or compression. On the basis of the arteriographic observations and the renal venous renin measurements (Table 1), a right nephrectomy was performed. After clamping of the right renal artery, the blood pressure decreased to 120/70. Two years after nephrectomy, the patient remained normotensive without medication.

Patient 2. The second patient was a 21-year-old white male who was referred to the Indiana University Medical Center for evaluation of hypertension of 6 months duration and a right renal mass on intravenous pyelography. He was first seen by his primary physician in April 1975 when he complained of persistent frontal headaches and was noted to have a blood pressure of 170/110. The patient had participated in athletics while in high school and had physical examinations with no mention of hypertension. There was also no history of renal or other serious disease. The only history of flank trauma that could be elicited was a fall while water skiing, which resulted in a minor back injury from hyperextension. The only family history of hypertension was some elevation of blood pressure during pregnancy in the patient's mother.

Physical examination after withdrawal of medication for 2 months revealed a blood pressure of 160/120. Examination of the ocular fundi showed only minimal arteriolar narrowing. There were no abdominal masses or abdominal bruits heard. The rest of the physical examination was negative. The laboratory studies were generally normal. The urinalysis was normal and the endogenous creatinine

TABLE 1. *Renal venous renin measurements (ng/ml 3 hr)*

Patient	Right renal vein	Inferior vena cava	Left renal vein
1			
Supine	270	26	23
45° Tilt	190	45	38
2			
Supine	90	64	64
45° Tilt	174	83	96

clearance was 92 ml/min. Both the chest X-ray and electrocardiogram were normal.

The renal arteriogram (Fig. 1) showed the left kidney to be normal in all respects. The right kidney had a dual vascular supply with both renal arteries patent. A large avascular mass was noted on the lateral aspect of the right kidney,

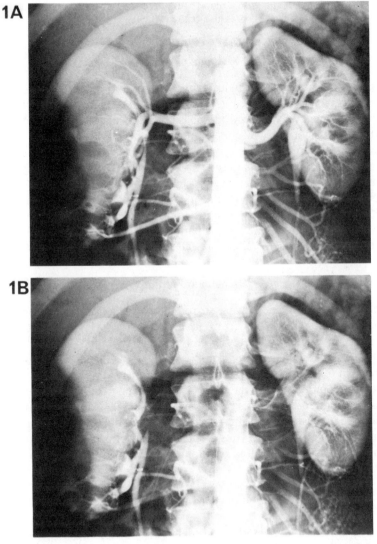

FIG. 1. Renal arteriogram in patient 2. **A.** Arterial phase with demonstration of the single left main renal artery and the dual arterial supply to the right kidney. Marked distortion and compression of the intrarenal vascular and collecting structures of the right kidney can be seen as well as the avascular area on the lateral aspect. **B:** Excretory phase further demonstrating distortion and medial displacement of the collecting system.

which caused compression of the adjacent parenchyma and medial distortion and compression of the pelvocalyceal system. This mass appeared to be subcapsular and spared both the most superior and inferior pole of the kidney.

Again, on the basis of the renal venous renin determinations (Table 1) and the arteriographic observations, surgery was performed. The blood pressure decreased to 118/80 with removal of the right kidney. At the time of discharge, the blood pressure was 130–125/90–85. On return visit 2 months later, a mild degree of hypertension was noted with a blood pressure of 140/90, which was treated with a diuretic to maintain blood pressure below 140/90.

Methods of Study

Plasma renin activity and aldosterone concentration were studied after a protocol previously described (3). These studies were also performed 3 months or more after surgery in the same subjects. Similar studies were performed in 13 normal white males aged 17 to 24 who served as controls. Plasma renin activity and aldosterone were measured by a previously described radioimmunoassay technique (11).

Renal venous renin samples were obtained following sodium depletion with a 10 meq sodium diet and furosemide in both the recumbent position and after 45° tilt for 20 min. The renal venous renin measurements are presented in Table 1. Prior to surgery, the second patient had a P-113[1] (Saralasin®) infusion to evaluate the response of blood pressure to this angiotensin antagonist (10).

Pathologic Findings

In both cases, the kidneys were surrounded by a dense fibrous capsule that enclosed approximately 200 cc of fluid in the cyst (Figs. 2 and 3). This structure involved nearly the entire convexity of the kidney but in both cases spared the hilar area. There was compression of the cortex and distortion and compression of the calyceal system in both patients. In neither case was there any evident compression of the renal artery. On microscopic examination of both kidneys, there were areas of fibrosis involving the superficial cortex with lymphocytic infiltration. Hyalinized glomeruli were observed in these areas as well as many normal appearing glomeruli. In both specimens, there was evidence of hyperplasia of the juxtaglomerular apparatus but none of arteriolar nephrosclerosis (Fig. 4).

RESULTS

The dynamic responses of plasma renin activity and aldosterone stimulation and suppression, for both patients before and after surgery, are compared to observations on normal subjects (Table 2). Both patients exhibited elevated plasma renin activity and plasma aldosterone after ambulation, and failed to

---

[1]Experimental drug: 1-sarc-8-ala angiotensin II.

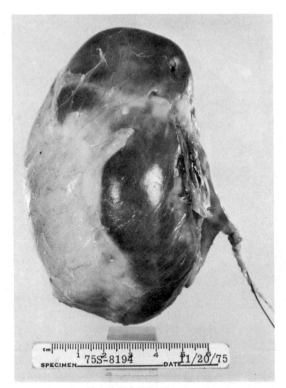

FIG. 2. Gross appearance of the right kidney in patient 2. Extensive perirenal fibrosis can be observed along the lateral aspect of the kidney, sparing most of the upper pole, part of the lower pole, and the hilar area. The subcapsular hematoma can be perceived medial to the area of fibrosis in the midportion of the kidney.

suppress plasma renin activity and plasma aldosterone appropriately after saline loading. They demonstrated marked stimulation of plasma renin activity after sodium and volume depletion. After surgery, both patients had lower values of plasma renin activity and plasma aldosterone at every point. In patient 1, these values were all within the normal range.

In patient 2, control blood pressure before P-113 was 148/108, and after 136/92. Three months after surgery the control blood pressure was 124/78 and after P-113, 118/68. In both patients, the blood pressure was markedly lower following nephrectomy. The first patient has remained normotensive for 2 years, whereas the second has mild hypertension easily controlled with a diuretic agent 6 months after surgery.

DISCUSSION

This study reports two patients with an unusual form of curable hypertension caused by constrictive fibrous encapsulation of the kidney, the "Page kidney." This form of hypertension has been produced experimentally by

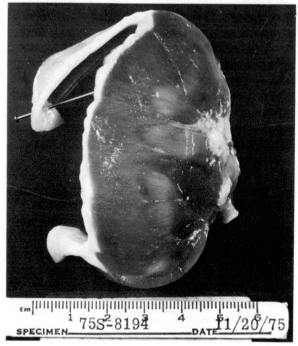

FIG. 3. Gross appearance of the sectioned kidney in patient 2. The dense fibrous capsule has been divided with a decrease in compression of the renal parenchyma. The lack of fibrosis at the extreme poles can also be appreciated as well as the compression of the collecting system.

TABLE 2. *Dynamic responses of renin and aldosterone*

| Subjects studied | Before saline | | After saline | | After furosemide |
	PRA (ng/ml/3 hr)	PA (ng/100 ml)	PRA	PA	PRA
Normal subjects (*n* = 13)					
Mean	6.1	33	1.2	5.6	33
(± SD)	(3.0)	(19)	(0.8)	(3.1)	(20)
Patient 1					
Before surgery	26	125	6.0	13.1	25
After surgery	7.4	44	0.8	2.2	26
Patient 2					
Before surgery	25	74	5.6	12.1	55
After surgery	12	103	2.3	8.1	52

PRA, plasma renin activity; PA, plasma aldosterone.

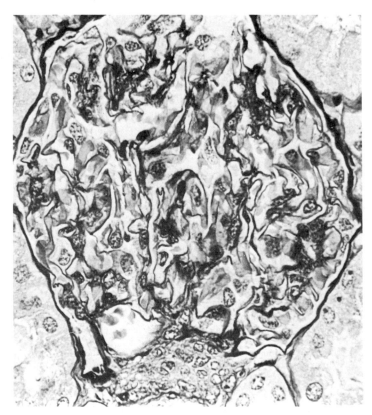

FIG. 4. Photomicrograph of a typical glomerulus in patient 1. The macula densa and juxta-glomerular area are at the midportion of the bottom of the figure and show increased granularity. ×400.

induction of perinephric inflammation and fibrosis secondary to enclosing the kidney in cellophane (6). Subsequent studies of this animal model have yielded contradictory results regarding the role of the renin-angiotensin system in the pathogenesis of the increase in blood pressure (1,4,5,7). The present study has demonstrated an abnormal stimulation of the renin-angiotensin-aldosterone that was restored to normal after surgery, elevation of renal venous renin activity from the involved kidney when compared to the contralateral kidney, microscopic evidence of increased juxtaglomerular granularity in the involved kidney tissue, and a significant decrease in blood pressure in the one patient to whom an angiotensin II antagonist, P-113, was administered. These studies thus indicate that this is a rare, but curable, form of hypertension that appears to be related to excessive and inappropriate renin production by the involved kidney. Finally, this form of hypertension should be considered in an individual with recent onset of hypertension, particularly if the individual is an active young male.

ACKNOWLEDGMENTS

The authors wish to express their gratitude to Ms. Mary B. Wade and Ms. Maria Ong for valuable technical assistance and to Ms. Gwendolyn L. Morgan for help in the preparation of this manuscript. We are also indebted to Drs. Fred Kuipers and Richard Pryor for recognizing the unusual patients described in this report and for permitting us to study them.

These studies were supported in part by USPHS Grant HL 14159, Specialized Center of Research in Hypertension.

REFERENCES

1. Campbell, D. J., Skinner, S. L., and Day, A. J. (1973): Cellophane perinephritis hypertension and its reversal in rabbits. *Circ. Res.,* 33:105–112.
2. Grim, C. E., Mullins, M. F., Nilson, J. P., and Ross, G., Jr. (1975): Unilateral "Page kidney" hypertension in man. JAMA, 231:42–45.
3. Grim, C. E., Weinberger, M. H., Kramer, N. J., and Higgins, J. T., Jr. (1975): A dynamic evaluation of the renin-aldosterone system in normals. *Clin. Res.,* 23:185A.
4. Lewis, P. J., and Lee, M. R. (1971): Plasma renin activity in the rabbit with renal hypertension. *Br. J. Exp. Pathol.,* 52:478–481.
5. Mogil, R. A., Itskovitz, H. D., Russell, J. H., and Russell, J. J. (1969): Renal innervation and renin activity in salt metabolism and hypertension. *Am. J. Physiol.,* 216:693–697.
6. Page, I. H. (1939): The production of persistent arterial hypertension by cellophane perinephritis. *JAMA,* 113:2046–2048.
7. Page, I. H. (1940): Demonstration of the liberation of renin into the blood stream from kidneys of animals made hypertensive by cellophane perinephritis. *Am. J. Physiol.,* 130:22–28.
8. Scott, P. L., Yune, H. Y., and Weinberger, M. H. (1976): An unusual cause of hypertension. *Radiol.,* 119:547–548.
9. Streeten, D. H. P., Anderson, G. H., Freiberg, J. M., and Dalakos, T. G. (1975): Use of an angiotensin II antagonist (Saralasin) in the recognition of "angiotensinogenic" hypertension. *N. Engl. J. Med.,* 292:657–662.
10. Sufrin, G. (1975): The Page kidney: A correctable form of arterial hypertension. *J. Urol.,* 113:450–454.
11. Weinberger, M. H., Kem, D. C., Gomez-Sanchez, C., Kramer, N. J., Martin, B. T., and Nugent, C. A. (1975): The effect of dexamethasone on the control of plasma aldosterone concentration in normal recumbent man. *J. Lab. Clin. Med.,* 85:957–967.

Juvenile Hypertension, edited by
M. I. New and L. S. Levine. Raven
Press, New York © 1977.

Comment: Syndromes of Hormonal Hypertension in Childhood

Lenore S. Levine

The uncoupling of the effect of aldosterone on urinary sodium, potassium, and hydrogen ion excretion was described by I. S. Edelman in the following comment: Aldosterone induces RNA and protein synthesis. The latent period for aldosterone effect on the urinary excretion of sodium, potassium, and hydrogen ions is the same, suggesting that the general mechanism of aldosterone effect is the same for these ions. However, the administration of actinomycin D, which inhibits RNA synthesis, produced varying effects:

(1) It blocks the sodium-retaining effect of aldosterone;
(2) decreases by 50% the potassium-excreting effect of aldosterone; and
(3) has no effect on the hydrogen ion excretion produced by aldosterone.

These effects suggest a possible mechanism for the dissociation of aldosterone effect on sodium, potassium, and hydrogen ions that may be observed.

Juvenile Hypertension, edited by
M. I. New and L. S. Levine. Raven
Press, New York © 1977.

An Unidentified ACTH-Stimulable Adrenal Steroid in Childhood Hypertension

Maria I. New and Lenore S. Levine

*Department of Pediatrics, The New York Hospital–Cornell Medical Center,
New York, New York 10021*

We would like to add to the body of data suggesting the existence of an unknown mineralocorticoid in low-renin hypertension.

In the clinical studies about to be presented, we have produced evidence that there is an ACTH-stimulable steroidal hormone capable of raising blood pressure. Furthermore, the data indicate that this steroidal hormone is not a *known* mineralocorticoid.

The first patient studied (E. M. G.) was an 18-year-old boy with dexamethasone-suppressible hyperaldosteronism and hypertension. He was first reported at the age of 12 years, and the subsequent studies indicated that aldosterone was the only steroid he oversecreted (1,2).

At age 18, the slightly elevated levels of urinary aldosterone were still readily suppressed with 1 mg of dexamethasone, although he rarely complied with medication at home (Fig. 1E).

With dexamethasone suppression, aldosterone excretion fell below 0.7 μg/day within 24 hr (Fig. 1F). The initially low renin (normal values 0.5 to 5 ng/ml/hr) rose as natriuresis occurred, accompanied by a slight weight loss. Blood pressure returned to normal over a period of 5 days. Urinary potassium decreased transiently. We reasoned that if aldosterone were causing the hypertension in the untreated state, then administration of aldosterone in the suppressed state should cause a rise in blood pressure.

With aldosterone excretion suppressed, and while the patient was normotensive, aldosterone was administered 1 mg i.v. daily over 24 hr for 5 days (Fig. 1G). This administration is reflected in the increased urinary excretion of aldosterone. Marked sodium retention and weight gain occurred but there was no significant change in blood pressure. There was slight kaliuresis and, inexplicably, plasma renin did not decrease, although 2 days later it was low. Thus, it appeared that aldosterone administration in large quantities induced sodium retention but *not* hypertension in this patient within a 5-day period.

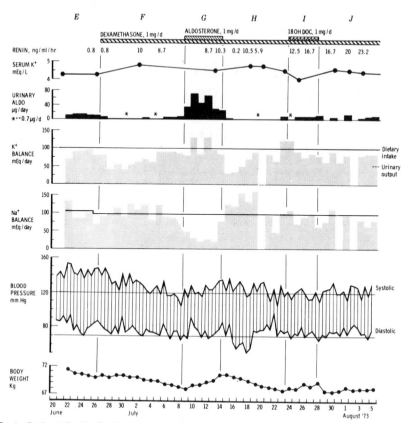

FIG. 1. Patient E. M. G. Metabolic balance of sodium and potassium correlated with blood pressure and various periods of therapy and hormonal measurements. This figure, as well as the others, depicts the medication, plasma renin activity, serum potassium, urinary aldosterone (pH 1), potassium balance, sodium balance, blood pressure, and weight. The blood pressure was taken six times during the day and six times during the night. The mean day and nighttime pressures are shown. (From New et al., ref. 2a.)

Aldosterone infusion was discontinued (Fig. 1H). The aldosterone excretion fell and natriuresis occurred with loss of body weight and potassium retention. The patient remained normotensive.

18-Hydroxydeoxycorticosterone (18-OH-DOC) was given, 1 mg i.v. over 24 hr for 5 days (Fig. 1I). Minimal changes in sodium and potassium balance occurred and there was no change in blood pressure. Low mineralocorticoid activity of 18-OH-DOC has been reported in bioassays (3–6). The unexplained high-renin levels were observed repeatedly. The failure of administered aldosterone and 18-OH-DOC to suppress renin may be the result of continuous dexamethasone suppression. Dexamethasone suppresses the ACTH-regulated aldosterone secretion, allowing plasma renin to rise, which then stimulates the renin-mediated aldosterone secretion. This mechanism has been described in 17-hydroxylase deficiency (7,8). No significant metabolic or blood pressure changes occurred when 18-OH-DOC administration ceased (Fig. 1J).

With continued dexamethasone treatment, deoxycorticosterone (DOC) was administered 30 mg i.v. daily for 5 days (Fig. 2K). A slight fall in serum potassium and increased urinary excretion of potassium occurred. There was marked sodium retention and a weight gain of 2 kg. Again, *no* increase in blood pressure was observed. Renin decreased somewhat but not to base-line levels. Failure of DOC to suppress plasma renin activity is unexplained. The effects of 30 mg administered DOC are similar to those of 1 mg administered aldosterone.

With discontinuation of DOC, natriuresis and potassium retention occurred, accompanied by a rise in serum potassium (Fig. 2L). The sodium retention, kaliuresis, and weight gain resulting from the administered DOC are validated by the reversal of the effect when DOC is discontinued. The lack of a DOC effect on blood pressure is also confirmed by the absence of change in blood pressure, whether or not the DOC was being administered. As was suggested for Fig. 2J, the continued excretion of small amounts of aldosterone suggests that the increased renin stimulates aldosterone despite ACTH suppression.

These studies of the effects of aldosterone, 18-OH-DOC, and DOC suggest that none of these hormones administered alone is capable of raising blood pressure after 5 days of continuous infusion, at superphysiological doses, despite a strong mineralocorticoid effect observed with aldosterone and DOC.

The next series of studies were designed in order to determine whether the 5-day period was too short to observe an effect of adrenal steroids on blood pressure.

After all treatment was discontinued, we wished to observe the length of time necessary for the patient's endogenous ACTH to reappear and produce hypertension and sodium retention (Fig. 2M). Within 5 days of discontinuing dexamethasone treatment, sodium retention and weight gain occurred. After 14 days without dexamethasone, urinary aldosterone excretion increased and plasma renin activity decreased after 7 days. However, hypertension did not recur even after 3 weeks without dexamethasone therapy, at a time when aldosterone excretion was high.

The dual regulation of aldosterone is again demonstrated in this period. After short-term dexamethasone suppression in this patient, aldosterone excretion decreased to below detectable levels, whereas renin remained suppressed, indicating ACTH regulation of aldosterone. It was shown in a previous report of this patient that (2), during dexamethasone treatment, a low-salt diet provoked a rise in renin and aldosterone in the dexamethasone-suppressed state. This renin regulation is again suggested at the end of prolonged dexamethasone suppression (Fig. 2L), when the renin remained elevated and aldosterone secretion was low but measurable. Two weeks following discontinuation of dexamethasone treatment, the urinary aldoste-

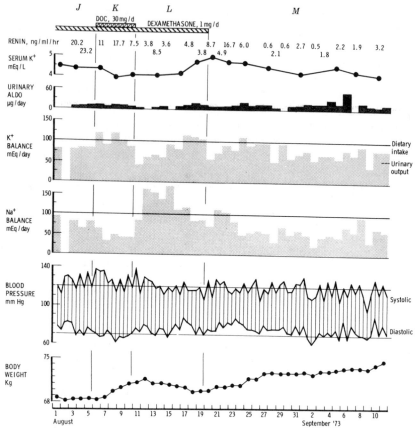

FIG. 2. Patient E. M. G. *See Fig. 1 legend for explanation.* (From New et al., ref. 2a.)

rone excretion increased and the plasma renin activity decreased. This suggests that ACTH regulation of aldosterone resumed by the 12th day after discontinuation of dexamethasone. Although aldosterone was being excreted in excess at the end of this period, hypertension did not recur, indicating that aldosterone did not raise blood pressure in this patient, even after 3 weeks of excess aldosterone secretion, sodium retention, and weight gain.

In order to evaluate whether infusion of ACTH was capable of producing an increase in blood pressure during the 5-day period of steroid infusion, ACTH (40 U i.v. over 24 hr for 6 days; 80 U i.v. over 24 hr for 2 days) was administered (Fig. 3N). This was associated with increased aldosterone excretion, sodium retention, weight gain, and a fall in serum potassium. The increased aldosterone excretion continued throughout the period of ACTH administration. The plasma renin activity did not decrease to the pretreatment levels observed in Fig. 1E.

The infusion of ACTH produced a rise in blood pressure within 5 days,

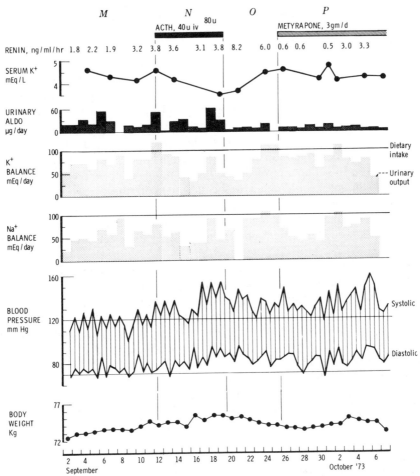

FIG. 3. Patient E. M. G. *See Fig. 1 legend for explanation.* (From New et al., ref. 2a.)

whereas infusion of aldosterone, 18-OH-DOC, or DOC administration was without effect on blood pressure in this period of time (Figs. 1 and 2; G, I, and K). This suggests that ACTH stimulated the adrenal secretion of a steroid other than that which was infused, and which was capable of causing a rise in blood pressure within 5 days. Quantitatively, the amount of aldosterone administered was far greater than that stimulated by the ACTH. Blood pressure, however, rose only during ACTH administration, further supporting the hypothesis that the blood pressure effect of ACTH was mediated through a hormone other than aldosterone. The failure of aldosterone to decrease during continuous ACTH administration was unexpected. Continuous ACTH administration has been reported to cause an initial increase in aldosterone excretion followed by a decrease within 5 days. The decrease is interpreted as "escape" from ACTH (9,10). Although sodium retention and weight gain were observed during ACTH, aldosterone, or DOC administration, plasma renin activity failed to decrease to the pretreatment levels observed in Fig. 1E.

The failure of ACTH to regularly induce a fall in renin has been reported by others (9,11). In addition, it has been demonstrated that DOC administration does not cause a decrease in plasma renin activity in subjects with various forms of hypertension (12), in contrast to the prompt decline observed in normal subjects when DOC is administered (13). This failure of DOC to suppress renin in hypertensive states has been attributed to the reduced cumulative sodium retention and weight gain in hypertensives as compared to normals (14). In patient E. M. G., however, renin suppression with mineralocorticoid administration failed to occur, even in the presence of sodium retention and weight gain. The response of renin to the administration of mineralocorticoids in hypertensives has not been studied extensively. Thus, the renin data in this patient as well as in other hypertensives remain to be clarified.

After ACTH was discontinued, aldosterone excretion decreased. Within 5 days, the patient returned to potassium and sodium balance (Fig. 3O). The patient lost 2 kg of weight, so that his weight was the same as that before the ACTH administration. Blood pressure decreased slightly. Plasma renin activity increased and serum potassium rose to 4.5 meq/liter. Thus, with discontinuation of ACTH, a rapid reversal of the mineralocorticoid effects was seen, although blood pressure changes were minimal.

Blood pressure had not returned to base-line levels at the start of metyrapone treatment. Administration of metyrapone produced a transient sodium retention and a marked fall in plasma renin activity (Fig. 4P). As sodium retention subsided, blood pressure and plasma renin activity increased. Aldosterone excretion remained low, but detectable, throughout the period of metyrapone treatment.

In this patient, blood pressure was maintained at an elevated level with metyrapone. It has been demonstrated that metyrapone interferes with the formation of cortisol by inhibiting the initial cleavage of cholesterol into pregnenolone, in addition to inhibiting the 11β-hydroxylation of 11-desoxycortisol (15). However, a compensatory ACTH increase can overcome the metyrapone inhibition of cholesterol side-chain cleavage activity (15). The rise in ACTH secretion in the presence of the 11β-hydroxylase inhibition results in a rise in DOC secretion. The elevation of blood pressure during metyrapone is probably not due to increased DOC secretion, because it was demonstrated (Fig. 2K) that 5 days of continuous DOC infusion in large amounts did not produce hypertension. The effects of metyrapone are probably secondary to increased secretion of ACTH. This is supported by the similar changes in weight, blood pressure, sodium and potassium balance, and plasma renin activity observed at the end of the ACTH and metyrapone treatment periods. The major difference between the ACTH (Fig. 3N) and metyrapone (Fig. 3P)

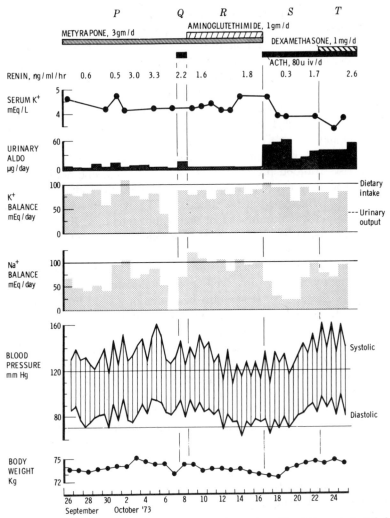

FIG. 4. Patient E. M. G. *See Fig. 1 legend for explanation.* (From New et al., ref. 2a.)

treatment is in the quantity of aldosterone excretion. During metyrapone administration, aldosterone excretion was not elevated. These studies further suggest that endogenous or exogenous ACTH can induce the adrenal secretion of an unidentified steroid capable of raising blood pressure. This unidentified hormone is not completely dependent on sodium retention for its capacity to raise blood pressure.

In order to determine whether ACTH mediates its effect on blood pressure, via secretion of a steroid hormone, or is in itself the blood pressure raising agent, metyrapone was continued and aminoglutethimide was added. The elevated blood pressure returned to normal, aldosterone excretion was markedly reduced, and a sodium diuresis and a rise in serum potassium ensued; body weight decreased slightly. Plasma renin activity remained at low-normal levels. Aminoglutethimide inhibits steroid synthesis by blocking the conversion of cholesterol to C_{21} steroids. ACTH secretion rises during aminoglutethimide treatment via the negative feedback adrenal–pituitary mechanism. The rapid fall in blood pressure to normal levels during this period is strong evidence that the hypertension observed during metyrapone (Fig. 3P) and ACTH administration (Fig. 3N) is caused by adrenal secretion of an unidentified steroid and not by a direct pressor action of ACTH.

Finally, ACTH was administered again, as before, with an even more dramatic rise in blood pressure, urinary aldosterone, and sodium retention (Fig. 4S). The hypertension was persistent, whereas the sodium retention was transient. Thus, the hypertensive effect of ACTH was reproducible (Fig. 3 and 4; N and S) and was not dependent on sodium retention. In both periods of ACTH administration, aldosterone excretion increased and remained elevated.

This failure of "escape" of aldosterone secretion from ACTH regulation is abnormal, and has been observed in hyperaldosteronism associated with adrenal hyperplasia (16). It has also been demonstrated in another kindred with dexamethasone-suppressible hyperaldosteronism (17).

The effect of ACTH was not diminished by concurrent administration of dexamethasone, demonstrating the dexamethasone treatment lowers blood pressure and aldosterone by suppressing ACTH and not by a peripheral action on the adrenals as suggested by Ruse et al. (18) (Fig. 4T).

We concluded from these studies that an ACTH-stimulable steroid other than aldosterone, 18-OH-DOC, or DOC may be the cause of hypertension in this patient. The metyrapone and aminoglutethimide studies further suggest that it is an adrenal steroid.

This hypothesis was strengthened by the study of a 3-year-old Zuni Indian girl (L. K.) (18a) with a 46/XX karyotype who presented with hypertension and hypokalemia. She had been hospitalized many times for gastroenteritis and survived without steroid treatment. The following studies were carried out in the Pediatric Clinical Research Center of the New York Hospital–Cornell Medical Center.

Urinary excretion of 17-ketosteroids, 17-hydroxysteroids, aldosterone, and morning plasma cortisol (4.9 μg/dl) were low (Fig. 5A). Hypokalemia was present and persisted despite potassium supplementation of 150 meq/day. Plasma renin activity was decreased (normal values 0.5 to 5 ng/ml/hr). Blood pressure was markedly elevated, and low-potassium intake at the end of this period resulted in decreased sodium wasting. Potassium has been shown to cause sodium wasting experimentally (20). Thus, this 3-year-old child demonstrated hypertension and hypokalemia in the absence of excessive aldosterone excretion.

A standard ACTH test (40 U i.v. over 6 hr) caused an increase in plasma

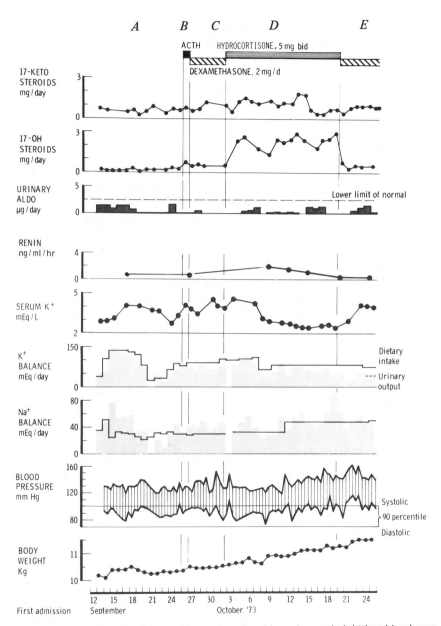

FIG. 5. Patient L. K. *See Fig. 1 legend for explanation.* Mean day- and nighttime blood pressures are presented. The 90th percentile blood pressure for a child of this age (3 years) (19) is indicated in each panel.

cortisol to 23 μg/dl (Fig. 5B). Urinary 17-hydroxysteroid excretion increased slightly when measured by the Porter-Silber chromogen method. Plasma renin activity remained low.

These findings suggest that the patient's capacity to secrete cortisol was impaired both in the base-line period and in response to ACTH. The low-plasma renin activity in the presence of low-urinary aldosterone, hypokalemia, and hypertension suggests the presence of a mineralocorticoid other than aldosterone.

Dexamethasone and hydrocortisone were administered sequentially (Fig. 5C, D, and E). The blood pressure did not decrease and, indeed, appeared to increase. The child became quite cushingoid and weight increased progressively. The 17-hydroxysteroids reflected the administration of hydrocortisone. Aldosterone excretion and plasma renin activity remained low.

While dexamethasone administration was continued, dietary sodium was reduced to 10 meq/day (Fig. 6F). This resulted in a negative sodium balance, and a prompt decrease in blood pressure. No change in weight or urinary aldosterone was observed. When potassium intake was reduced from 60 to 30 meq/day, a marked decrease in urinary sodium occurred. Despite the decreased potassium intake, she remained in positive potassium balance and serum potassium rose.

The fall in blood pressure upon restriction of dietary sodium demonstrates the dependence of blood pressure on sodium intake. This decrease in blood pressure occurred despite the continuation of dexamethasone treatment that had previously caused elevation of blood pressure. The ability to conserve sodium in the absence of an elevation of urinary aldosterone suggests the presence of another mineralocorticoid. Her capacity to conserve sodium as well as potassium indicated good renal function. The fall in blood pressure observed in the absence of weight loss suggests there was not net fluid loss.

Blood pressure and serum potassium remained in the normal range when dexamethasone was discontinued (Fig. 6G). Plasma renin activity as well as urinary aldosterone excretion remained low at the end of this period and after 15 days of dietary sodium restriction (10 meq/day).

We interpreted these results to mean that the important element in the fall in blood pressure was the sodium restriction; dexamethasone did not contribute to the fall in blood pressure. The absence of weight loss when blood pressure was reduced indicates that the sodium effect was not mediated through a measurable loss of body water. The persistent suppression of plasma renin activity despite dietary sodium restriction suggests that a mineralocorticoid was present. The effect of the unknown mineralocorticoid on blood pressure, however, was not apparent in the sodium-restricted state.

While the low-sodium diet was maintained, ACTH was administered (40 U/day i.v.) continuously for 5 days (Fig. 6H). Urinary 17-ketosteroids and 17-hydroxycorticoids rose to 2 and 7 mg/day, respectively, but aldosterone

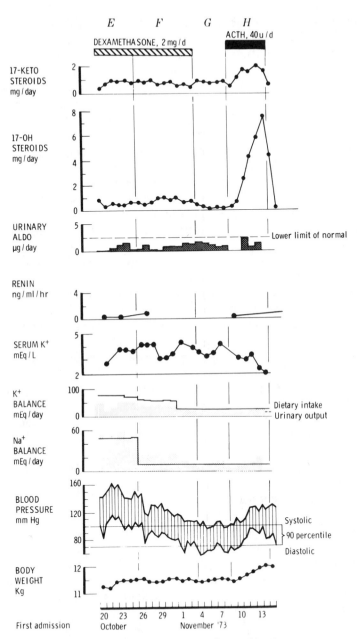

FIG. 6. Patient L. K. *See Fig. 1 for explanation.*

excretion never increased above 2 μg/day. Plasma cortisol rose to a maximum of 32 μg/dl. Serum potassium concentration fell to less than 2 meq/liter. Blood pressure increased significantly and there was a 0.5 kg gain in weight. Urinary sodium and potassium excretion did not change from the pre-ACTH period.

Thus, an increase in blood pressure was produced by ACTH without a concomitant increase in aldosterone excretion. This suggests that ACTH stimulated a factor, other than aldosterone, that is capable of raising blood pressure. This factor appears to be a mineralocorticoid, as is evident by the precipitous fall in serum potassium concentration. The fall in serum potassium was apparently not the result of kaliuresis, as no increase in urinary potassium was observed. The weight gain suggests fluid retention despite the low-sodium intake. The ability of ACTH to increase blood pressure was sufficient to override the hypotensive effect of a low-sodium diet. Blood pressure was restored to hypertensive levels observed on a normal sodium diet. Thus, the factor stimulated by ACTH, which raises blood pressure, is only partly dependent on sodium intake. The rise in 17-hydroxycorticoid excretion and plasma cortisol suggests that the adrenal is capable of secreting glucocorticoids but not to a normal degree. Children of similar size and age increase urinary 17-hydroxycorticoids to 60 mg/day and plasma cortisol to 70 μg/dl after 5 days of ACTH (*unpublished data*). Thus, it seems likely that ACTH was stimulating a hormone that is a mineralocorticoid capable of raising blood pressure and that may be the same hormone causing hypertension, hypokalemia, and hyporeninemia in the untreated state. The failure of ACTH to stimulate aldosterone, even transiently, shows a marked defect in aldosterone secretion. The subnormal increase in urinary 17-hydroxycorticoids and plasma cortisol with prolonged ACTH treatment indicates that glucocorticoid secretion is also impaired, but to a lesser extent, than aldosterone.

With discontinuation of ACTH, blood pressure decreased within 48 hr (Fig. 7I). Urinary 17-hydroxycorticoids and 17-ketosteroids fell promptly to low-pretreatment levels. Weight declined slightly. Serum potassium rose after ACTH had been discontinued for 5 days; aldosterone excretion did not change significantly.

Throughout the entire study, aldosterone excretion and plasma renin activity remained low and fairly fixed. The rise in 17-hydroxysteroids and plasma cortisol with ACTH and the rapid fall when ACTH was discontinued raises the possibility that in the untreated state ACTH is suppressed by an unidentified steroid, resulting in a very low glucocorticoid secretion (see plasma ACTH concentration below).

When potassium intake was increased to 100 meq/day, blood pressure did not change significantly (Fig. 7J). There was net potassium retention and a rise in serum potassium to 4.5 meq/liter. Aldosterone excretion and plasma renin activity remained at low levels. There was a slight weight gain and natriuresis occurred. Although administration of large amounts of potassium is recog-

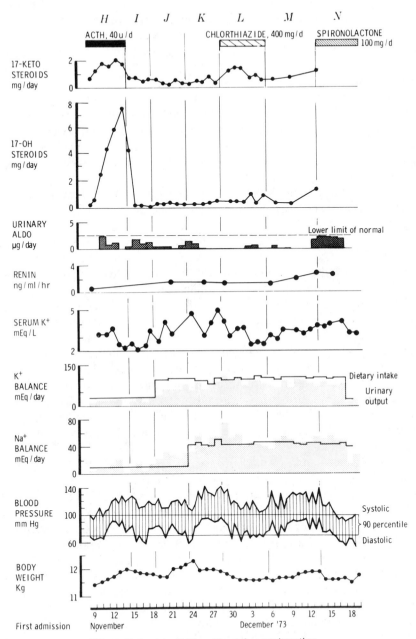

FIG. 7. Patient L. K. *See Fig. 1 for explanation.*

nized as a potent stimulator of aldosterone secretion in both normal subjects and those with hyperaldosteronism, the stimulus did not produce any increase in aldosterone in this patient. Renin was also not stimulated despite a natriuresis in association with a high-potassium intake. The effect of dietary sodium restriction in lowering the blood pressure persisted.

With an increase in dietary sodium to normal amounts for age (40 meq/day) (Fig. 7K), the blood pressure rose to the hypertensive levels observed prior to initiation of the low-sodium diet; serum potassium fluctuated. Urinary excretion of 17-hydroxysteroids, aldosterone, and plasma renin activity did not change significantly. It appears, therefore, that in this child blood pressure is responsive to both ACTH and sodium.

Administration of chlorothiazide (400 mg/day) produced a transient natriuresis, a fall in blood pressure to normal limits, and a weight loss of 0.5 kg (Fig. 7L). A decrease in serum potassium ensued without kaliuresis. Urinary excretion of aldosterone and 17-hydroxysteroids and plasma renin activity remained low. The effect of chlorothiazide to decrease blood pressure is probably mediated via the natriuretic effect. Although natriuresis is usually a stimulus to renin and aldosterone, the failure of these parameters to increase under provocative conditions was again demonstrated.

Discontinuation of chlorothiazide resulted in a rise in blood pressure and weight increase of 0.5 kg (Fig. 7M). A rise in serum potassium concentration to 3.6 meq/liter was associated with potassium retention. The capacity of normal dietary sodium to raise blood pressure was again demonstrated. The fact that the decrease in blood pressure produced by chlorothiazide was mediated by the natriuresis is supported by the rise in blood pressure when natriuresis ended. The changes in weight were not as marked as changes in blood pressure. The known kaliuretic and hypokalemic effect of chlorothiazide makes it an unlikely therapeutic modality in this child.

Spironolactone administration produced a prompt fall in blood pressure without significant change in urinary aldosterone (Fig. 7N). Serum potassium concentration rose. Plasma renin activity was slightly higher but appeared to have risen before spironolactone was administered. There was a slight natriuresis and a weight gain of 0.5 kg. Since spironolactone blocks mineralocorticoid action in the kidney, the fall in blood pressure and the normalization of serum potassium concentration with spironolactone strongly suggests that this patient secretes a mineralocorticoid capable of raising blood pressure and causing hypokalemia. This mineralocorticoid is not aldosterone because aldosterone was not secreted in significant quantities in this patient. The capacity of spironolactone to lower blood pressure distinguishes this patient from those described by Liddle et al. (21) who responded to triamterene and not to spironolactone. Spironolactone is a good therapeutic drug in this patient because it lowered blood pressure and corrected the hypokalemia.

The secretion rates of desoxycortisol, cortisol, desoxycorticosterone, corticosterone, and aldosterone were low in the base-line period. This patient had a surface area of 0.5 m², and the normal data are given for comparison (Table 1) (22). With ACTH stimulation, there was a slight increase to still subnormal levels in the patient. With dexamethasone, the secretion rates of both the normal subjects and those of the patient were extremely low.

The ACTH level on the morning of her seventh day of admission—September 18, 1973 (Fig. 5A)—was less than 50 pg/ml, as measured by Yalow (23). At this level, low and normal values cannot be distinguished, but it is clear that the level is not elevated in this patient. The absence of elevated ACTH levels in the presence of low cortisol secretion rate, low 17-hydroxycorticoid excretion, and low plasma cortisol suggests a factor other than cortisol that suppresses ACTH. If the ACTH level were low, it would explain the low secretion of all the steroids measured. Since the patient does respond to administered ACTH, albeit sluggishly, it is apparent that the adrenal has the capacity to secrete these hormones. Indeed, with prolonged ACTH administration (Fig. 6H), there is a significant rise in the excretion of 17-hydroxycorticoids, which suggests a significant increase in the secretion rate of adrenal hormones at this time.

A steroid recently suggested to be important in low-renin hypertension, 16-hydroxydehydroepiandrosterone (16-OH-DHEA) (24), was very low in this patient's urine (Table 2). Other steroids of interest in low-renin hypertension were also low (25–27).

DISCUSSION

The evidence for secretion of an unknown adrenocortical steroid in low-renin hypertension has been recently summarized by Liddle and co-workers (28). Various mineralocorticoids have been implicated in low-renin hypertension. A role for DOC in the etiology of low-renin hypertension may be speculated on because DOC is secreted in excess in certain hypertensive

TABLE 1. *Adrenal hormone secretion rates (mg/day)*

	B	S	F	DOC	Aldosterone
Base line					
Normal adult	3.8	0.38	11.5	0.085	0.18
Normal adult/m²	2.0	0.26	7.5	0.055	0.13
Normal child/0.5 m²	1.2	0.13	3.8	0.025	0.02–1.6
L. K.	0.057	0.06	0.04	0.026	0.02
ACTH (1 day)					
Normal child/0.5 m²	5.0	10.0	12.0	0.2	0.100
L. K.	0.21	0.22	1.4	0.068	0.013
Dexamethasone					
Normal adult/0.5 m²	< 1	< 1	< 1	< 1	0.04
L. K.	0.03	0.05	0.04	0.027	0.005

B, corticosterone; S, 11-deoxycortisol; F, cortisol.

TABLE 2. *Excretion of steroid metabolites of interest in low-renin hypertension*

Urinary steroids (μg/day)	L. K.	Normal adult	Normal child	Reference to normal range
16β-OH-DHEA	7.8	19–116	—	25
3β,17β-Dihydroxy-5-androsten-16-one	83.0	60–360	—	25
18-OH-tetrahydro-DOC	< 4	15	—	57
18-OH-tetrahydroaldosterone	< 4	122 ± 35	39 ± 21	27
Tetrahydroaldosterone	< 4	53 ± 20	19 ± 9	27

(Reproduced from Ulick, ref. 57.)

states (7,8,22). DOC administration has produced hypertension (14,29–34), and elevated plasma DOC concentrations have been found in some patients with low-renin hypertension (35). The role of aldosterone in the production of hypertension is less clear, although hyperaldosteronism is associated with certain hypertensive disorders (36). Administration of aldosterone to humans has produced strong mineralocorticoid effects, but variable effects on blood pressure (37–41). Two studies showed no change in blood pressure (37,41); one did not mention blood pressure (38) and the two studies carried out by August et al. (39,40) showed a rise in blood pressure when maximal weight gain occurred at the end of 26 days of aldosterone administration. The other studies cited here (37,38,41) administered aldosterone for a maximum of 10 days. Thus, the variable effects on blood pressure may be influenced by the duration of aldosterone administration. The role of 18-OH-DOC in hypertension remains controversial (42–44).

In the first patient (E. M. G.), in whom the only steroid known to be oversecreted was aldosterone, remission of hypertension occurred when aldosterone was suppressed by dexamethasone. We have documented, however, that aldosterone is not the ACTH-stimulable hormone that produced hypertension within 5 days. ACTH, when given to either normal individuals or patients with hyperaldosteronism, has been shown to produce a transient increase in aldosterone secretion or excretion but no change in plasma renin (9). In patients, including those with hyperaldosteronism, aldosterone excretion returned to unstimulated levels by the third day of ACTH administration. The same phenomenon of the transient ACTH effect on aldosterone excretion has been observed by others (10,45,46), which is in contrast to the persistent stimulation of aldosterone by ACTH in this patient.

Although hypertension is common in Cushing's syndrome (47), and is frequently associated with steroid administration (48), the role of hypercortisolemia in the etiology of hypertension is obscure. Of interest, is the greater incidence of hypertension that is found with chronically administered ACTH than with corticosteroids (49), suggesting that a steroid other than cortisol may be responsible for the hypertension. The effect of ACTH administration on blood pressure in man has not received great attention.

In the first patient (E. M. G.), the data suggest that a patient with dexamethasone-suppressible hyperaldosteronism secretes an adrenal steroid, induced by ACTH, that is not a known mineralocorticoid. Although we have not identified the steroid, we have demonstrated that neither aldosterone, 18-OH-DOC, nor DOC administered alone produces hypertension within 5 days, which is in contrast to the rapid hypertensive effect of ACTH administration. We did not, however, administer steroids in combination as was done in sheep (50). The pressor effect of 5 days of metyrapone and the absence of the pressor effect of 5 days of DOC administration in this patient suggests that the ACTH-induced hypertensive steroid is an 11-desoxysteroid other than DOC.

Further studies using blood and urine collected under ACTH and metyrapone stimulation may provide a source from which we may characterize this steroid.

The second patient (L. K.) provides the most persuasive evidence for the presence of an unidentified ACTH-stimulable hormone that has both mineralocorticoid and glucocorticoid activity and is capable of raising blood pressure. This patient manifests strong mineralocorticoid effects and hypertension in the absence of excessive secretion of any known sodium-retaining steroid. The mineralocorticoid activity of this hormone is reflected in the hypokalemia and suppressed renin in the untreated state and the aggravation of the hypokalemia with ACTH administration. The glucocorticoid effect is suggested by the lack of elevation of plasma ACTH in the presence of low 17-hydroxycorticoid excretion, plasma cortisol, and cortisol secretion. Further evidence for glucocorticoid activity is provided by the ability of the patient to survive repeated episodes of severe gastroenteritis, including *Salmonella sepsis,* without glucocorticoid replacement despite low secretion and excretion of cortisol.

The pressor effect of this unknown hormone is evident in the hypertension in the untreated state, which increased after ACTH administration. Although the pressor effect of the ACTH-stimulable hormone showed sodium dependence, administration of ACTH apparently overrode the hypotensive effect of low-sodium diet.

Hypertension that is produced in sheep following administration of ACTH (11,50) is in some ways similar to that observed in the patient L. K. Both are hypokalemic, hypertensive states that persist even on a low-sodium intake, and can occur without changes in weight and external electrolyte balance. In both, the hypertensive effect of ACTH can be observed on a low-sodium intake. The known components of the sheep's adrenocortical effluent, including 18-OH-DOC when reinfused, did not reproduce the hypertension within 24 hr as did the administration of ACTH (50). In a recent preliminary report, Scoggins et al. (51) indicated that the steroid $17\alpha,20\alpha$-dihydroxy-4-pregnen-3-one in the sheep's adrenal vein blood is capable of reproducing the rapid hypertensive effect of ACTH when administered along with the known adrenal secretory components.

Several cases of apparent mineralocorticoid excess have been described in which the patients are hypertensive and hypokalemic but the aldosterone secretion is very low. The first study was that of Liddle et al. (21) who described eight patients in a kindred who had severe hypertension and hypokalemia that was resistent to treatment with spironolactone or low-sodium diet. Treatment with triamterene reduced blood pressure and caused a rise in serum potassium when dietary sodium was decreased. Other cases with similar findings have been described (52–55). One of these cases responded to spironolactone (54), while another required triamterene (55).

The patient whose disorder most closely resembled that of patient L. K. was described by Werder et al. (56). Werder's patient was also a 3-year-old female with low-excretion of glucocorticoids and mineralocorticoids. In his case, the most important difference appeared to be the rise in renin and aldosterone that was caused by salt restriction and spironolactone. Werder and co-workers also proposed an unknown steroid with mineralocorticoid and glucocorticoid activity as the best explanation for all the features, including a low-normal ACTH level.

In summary, we have presented a case of apparent mineralocorticoid excess in a 3-year-old girl. The features are hypertension, hypokalemia, hyporeninemia, and reduced-to-absent secretion of mineralocorticoids and glucocorticoids. The data suggest the presence of an as yet unidentified hormone that is stimulated by ACTH and that has both mineralocorticoid and glucocorticoid activity. The pressor effect of the hormone is partly dependent on sodium. The hypertension and hypokalemia are improved with spironolactone treatment.

The patients L. K. and E. M. G. provide strong evidence for an unidentified ACTH-stimulable adrenal steroid that plays an important role in certain forms of low-renin hypertension. It would seem important to characterize this steroid and investigate its role in other forms of hypertension.

ACKNOWLEDGMENTS

This investigation was supported in part by USPHS, NIH Grants HE 12239, HL 17749, HD 00072, and HL 18323; USPHS, NIH Division of Research Facilities and Resources, Clinical Research Centers RR 47; and the National Foundation–March of Dimes Awards CRBS 278 and 6-75170.

REFERENCES

1. New, M. I., and Peterson, R. E. (1967): A new form of congenital adrenal hyperplasia. *J. Clin. Endocrinol. Metab.*, 27:300–305.
2. New, M. I., Siegal, E., and Peterson, R. E. (1973): Dexamethasone-suppressible hyperaldosteronism. *J. Clin. Endocrinol. Metab.*, 37:93–100.
2a. New, M. I., Peterson, R. E., Saenger, P., and Levine, L. S. (1976): Evidence for an

unidentified ACTH-induced steroid hormone causing hypertension. *J. Clin. Endocrinol. Metab.*, 43:1283–1293.

3. Melby, J. C., Dale, S. L., Greikin, R. J., Gaunt, R., and Wilson, T. E. (1972): 18-Hydroxy-11-deoxycorticosterone (18-OH-DOC) secretion in experimental and human hypertension. *Recent Prog. Horm. Res.*, 28:287–351.

4. Kagawa, C. M., and Pappo, R. (1962): Renal electrolyte effects of synthetic 18-hydroxylated steroids in adrenalectomized rats. *Proc. Soc. Exp. Biol. Med.*, 109:982–985.

5. Gotshall, R. W., and Davis, J. O. (1973): Mineralocorticoid activity of 18-hydroxydeoxycorticosterone in the dog. *Am. J. Physiol.*, 224:1116–1118.

6. Porter, G. A., and Kimsey, J. (1971): Assessment of the mineralocorticoid activity of 18-hydroxydeoxycorticosterone (18-OH-DOC) in the isolated toad bladder. *Endocrinology*, 89:353–357.

7. New, M. I. (1971): Male pseudohermaphroditism due to 17-hydroxylase deficiency. *J. Clin. Invest.*, 49:1930–1941.

8. Biglieri, E. G., Herron, M. A., and Brust, N. (1966): 17-Hydroxylation deficiency in man. *J. Clin. Invest.*, 45:1946–1954.

9. Newton, M. A., and Laragh, J. H. (1968): Effect of corticotropin on aldosterone excretion and plasma renin in normal subjects, in essential hypertension and in primary aldosteronism. *J. Clin. Endocrinol. Metab.*, 28:1006–1013.

10. Biglieri, E. G., Shambelan, M., and Slaton, P. E., Jr. (1969): Effect of adrenocorticotropin on desoxycorticosterone, corticosterone and aldosterone excretion. *J. Clin. Endocrinol. Metab.*, 29:1090–1101.

11. Scoggins, B. A., Coughlan, C. P., Denton, D. A., Fan, J. S. K., McDougall, J. G., Oddie, C. J., and Shulkes, A. A. (1974): Metabolic effects of ACTH in the sheep. *Am. J. Physiol.*, 226:198–205.

12. Biglieri, E. G., Schambelan, M., and Stockigt, J. R. (1972): The effect of desoxycorticosterone acetate (DOCA) on aldosterone and plasma renin activity (PRA) levels in hypertension and hyperaldosteronism. In: *Proceedings of IV International Congress on Endocrinology*, Washington, D. C., p. 109. (Abstract #271).

13. Shade, R. E., and Grim, C. E. (1975): Suppression of renin and aldosterone by small amounts of DOCA in normal man. *J. Clin. Endocrinol. Metab.*, 40:652–658.

14. Biglieri, E. G., Schambelan, M., Slaton, P. E., and Stockigt, J. R. (1970): The intercurrent hypertension of primary aldosteronism. *Circ. Res.*, 26,27(Suppl. I):1–195.

15. Carballeira, A., Fishman, L. M., and Jacobi, J. D. (1976): Dual sites of inhibition by metyrapone of human adrenal steroidogenesis: Correlation of in vivo and in vitro studies. *J. Clin. Endocrinol. Metab.*, 42:687–695.

16. Miura, K., Yoshinaga, K., Goto, K., Katsushima, I., Maebashi, M., Demura, H., Iino, M., Demura, R., and Toriki, T. (1968): A case of glucocorticoid-responsive hyperaldosteronism. *J. Clin. Endocrinol. Metab.*, 28:1807–1815.

17. Grim, C. E., Weinberger, M. H., Anand, S. K., and Northway, J. D. (1975): Familial, normokalemic glucocorticoid suppressible hyperaldosteronism. In: *Proceedings of VI International Congress on Nephrology*, Florence, Italy. (Abstract #605).

18. Ruse, J. L., Price, C., Stiefel, M., and Laidlaw, J. C. (1972): The influence of glucocorticoids and heparin on aldosterone production. In: *Hypertension '72*, edited by J. Genest and E. Koiw, pp. 326–333. Springer-Verlag, Berlin.

18a. New, M. I., Levine, L. S., Biglieri, E. G., Pareira, J., and Ulick, S. (1977): Evidence for an unidentified steroid in a child with apparent mineralocorticoid hypertension. *J. Clin. Endocrinol. Metab., in press*.

19. McCammon, R. W. (ed.) (1970): Vital signs—blood pressure—pulse. In: *Human Growth and Development*, pp. 49–59. Charles C Thomas, Springfield, Ill.

20. Brandis, M., Keyes, J., and Windhager, E. E. (1972): Potassium-induced inhibitors of proximal tubular fluid resorption in rats. *Am. J. Physiol.*, 222:421–427.

21. Liddle, G. W., Bledsoe, T., and Coppage, W. S. (1963): A familial renal disorder simulating primary aldosteronism but with negligible aldosterone secretion. *Trans. Assoc. Am. Physicians*, 76:199.

22. New, M. I., and Seaman, M. P. (1970): Secretion rates of cortisol and aldosterone precursors in various forms of congenital adrenal hyperplasia. *J. Clin. Endocrinol. Metab.*, 30:361–371.

23. Berson, S. P., and Yalow, R. S. (1968): Radioimmunoassay of ACTH and plasma. *J. Clin. Invest.*, 477:2725–2751.
24. Liddle, G. W., and Sennet, J. A. (1975): New mineralocorticoids in the syndrome of low-renin essential hypertension. *J. Steroid. Biochem.*, 6:751–753.
25. Jänne, O., and Vihko, R. (1969): Monosulfates of 16-oxygenated ketonic C19 steroids in adult human urine. *Steroids*, 14:235–250.
26. Melby, J. C., Dale, S. L., Grekin, R. J., Gaunt, R., and Wilson, T. E. (1972): 18-Hydroxy-11-deoxycorticosterone (18-OH-DOC) secretion in essential and human hypertension. In: *Hypertension '72*, edited by J. Genest and E. Koiw, p. 350. Springer-Verlag, Berlin.
27. Ulick, S. (1976): Diagnosis and nomenclature of the disorders of the terminal portion of the aldosterone biosynthetic pathway. *J. Clin. Endocrinol. Metab.*, 43:92–96.
28. Liddle, G. W., Carey, R. M., and Douglas, J. G. (1973): Role of the adrenal cortex in the pathogenesis of essential hypertension with suppressed renin. In: *International Congress Series 273*, pp. 752–756. Excerpta Medica, Amsterdam.
29. Luft, R., Sjögren, B., Ikkos, D., Ljunggren, H., and Tarukoski, H. (1954): Clinical studies on electrolyte and fluid metabolism. Effect of ACTH, desoxycorticosterone acetate and cortisone: Electrolyte and fluid changes in acromegaly. *Recent Prog. Horm. Res.*, 10:425–470.
30. Vagnucci, A. H., and Shapiro, A. P. (1974): Perspectives on the renin-angiotensin-aldosterone system in hypertension. *Metabolism.* 23:273–302.
31. Perera, G. A., Knowlton, A. I., Lowell, A., and Loeb, R. F. (1944): Effect of desoxycorticosterone acetate on the blood pressure of man. *JAMA*, 125:1030–1035.
32. Perera, G. A. (1948): Effect of continued desoxycorticosterone administration in hypertensive subjects. *Proc. Soc. Exp. Biol. Med.*, 68:48–50.
33. Ferrebee, J. W., Ragan, C., Atchley, D. W., and Loeb, R. F. (1939): Desoxycorticosterone esters. Certain effects in the treatment of Addison's disease. *JAMA*, 113:1725–1731.
34. Soffer, L. J., Engle, F. L., and Oppenheimer, B. S. (1940): Treatment of Addison's disease with desoxycorticosterone acetate. *JAMA*, 115:1860–1866.
35. Brown, J. J., Fraser, R., Love, D. R., Ferris, J. B., Lever, A. F., Robertson, J. I., and Wilson, A. (1972): Apparently isolated excess deoxycorticosterone in hypertension. A variant of the mineralocorticoid-excess syndrome. *Lancet*, 2:243–247.
36. Ross, E. J. (1975): *Aldosterone and Aldosteronism.* Lloyd-Luke, Ltd., London.
37. Rosemberg, E., Demany, M., Budnitz, E., Underwood, R., Leard, A., and Leard, R. S. (1962): Effects of administration of large amounts of d-aldosterone in normal subjects and in a patient with Sheenan's syndrome. *J. Clin. Endocrinol. Metab.*, 22:465–480.
38. Ross, E. J., and Hurst, P. E. (1965): Effect of prolonged administration of aldosterone and corticosterone on plasma and urinary electrolytes in man. *Clin. Sci.*, 28:91–98.
39. August, J. T., Nelson, D. H., and Thorn, G. W. (1958): Response of normal subjects to large amounts of aldosterone. *J. Clin. Invest.*, 37:1549–1555.
40. August, J. T., and Nelson, D. H. (1959): Adjustment to aldosterone or desoxycorticosterone acetate induced sodium retention in patients with Addison's disease. *J. Clin. Invest.*, 38:1964–1971.
41. Dawborn, J. K. (1969): The effect of prolonged intraveneous infusion of aldosterone in a normal human subject. *Med. J. Australia*, 1:1079–1083.
42. Ulick, S. (1973): Normal and alternate pathways in aldosterone synthesis. *International Congress Series 273*, pp. 761–767. Excerpta Medica, Amsterdam.
43. Genest, J., Nowacyznski, W., Kuchel, O., and Sasaki, C. (1972): Plasma progesterone levels and 18-hydroxydeoxycorticosterone secretion rate in benign essential hypertension in humans. In: *Hypertension '72*, edited by J. Genest and E. Koiw, p. 293. Springer-Verlag, New York.
44. Messerli, F. H., Kuchel, O., Nowaczynski, W., Seth, K., Honda, M., Kubo, S., Boucher, R, Tolis, G., and Genest, J. (1976): Mineralocorticoid secretion in essential hypertension with normal and low plasma renin activity. *Circulation*, 53:406–410.
45. Dluhy, R. G., and Williams, G. H. (1969): Primary aldosteronism in a hypertensive acromegalic patient. *J. Clin. Endocrinol. Metab.*, 29:1319–1324.
46. Slaton, P. E., Jr., Schambelan, M., and Biglieri, E. G. (1969): Stimulation and suppression of aldosterone secretion in patients with an aldosterone-producing adenoma. *J. Clin. Endocrinol. Metab.*, 29:239–250.

47. Plotz, C. M., Knowlton, A. I., and Ragan, C. (1952): The natural history of Cushing's syndrome. *Am. J. Med.,* 13:597–614.
48. Ragan, C. (1953): Corticotropin, cortisone and related steroids in clinical medicine: Practical considerations. *Bull. N.Y. Acad. Med.,* 29:355–376.
49. Savage, O., Copeman, W. S., Chapman, L., Wells, M. V., and Treadwell, B. L. (1962): Pituitary and adrenal hormones in rheumatoid arthritis, *Lancet,* 1:232–235.
50. Fan, J. S. K., Coghlan, J. P., Denton, D. A., Oddie, C. J., Scoggins, B. A., and Shulkes, A. A. (1975): Effect of intravenous infusion of corticosteroids on blood pressure, electrolytes and water metabolism in sheep. *Am. J. Physiol.,* 228:1695–1701.
51. Scoggins, B. A., Coghlan, J. P., Denton, D. A., Fan, J. S., and McDougall, J. G. (1976): Mechanism of ACTH induced hypertension. In: *Program and Abstracts—58th Annual Meeting, The Endocrine Society,* San Francisco, Calif. (Abstract #211).
52. Aarskog, D., Støa, K. F., Thorsen, T., and Wefring, K. W. (1967): Hypertension and hypokalemia alkalosis with underproduction of aldosterone. *Pediatrics,* 39:884–890.
53. Ross, E. J. (1959): Hypertension and hypokalemia associated with hypoaldosteronism. *Proc. Royal Soc. Med.,* 2:1056.
54. Ross, E. J. (1975): *Aldosterone and Aldosteronism,* p. 306. Lloyd-Luke, Ltd., London.
55. Milora, R., Vagnucci, A., and Goodman, A. D. (1967): A syndrome resembling primary aldosteronism but without mineralocorticoid excess (MCE). *Clin. Res.,* 15:482.
56. Werder, E., Zachmann, M., Völlman, J. A., Veyrat, R., and Prader, A. (1973): Unusual steroid excretion in a child with low-renin hypertension. *International Study Group for Steroid Hormones.* Rome, Dec. (Abstract).
57. Ulick, S. (1976): Adrenocortical factors in hypertension: The significance of 18-hydroxy-11-deoxycorticosterone. *Am. J. Med., in press.*

[1]Portions of this chapter are reproduced with the permission of the publisher J. B. Lippincott Co., and the editors of *J. Clin. Endocrinol. Metab.,* 1976, Vol. 43, *in press.*

Juvenile Hypertension, edited by
M. I. New and L. S. Levine. Raven
Press, New York © 1977.

Steroid Patterns in a Juvenile Hypertensive Syndrome

Stanley Ulick and Leyla C. Ramirez

Veterans Administration Hospital, Bronx, New York 10468

The findings in the second of the two patients described by New and Levine (1) strongly suggested the secretion of an unknown mineralocorticoid. This report describes our efforts to define an adrenocortical abnormality in that patient (L. K.) whose clinical and laboratory findings resembled those of primary aldosteronism, except that the production of aldosterone and other known steroids was subnormal.

Proceeding on the assumption that an adrenocortical abnormality would be reflected in an abnormal steroid pattern, the following studies were carried out.

PROCEDURES TO DETECT ADRENOCORTICAL ABNORMALITY

Analysis of Urinary Fractions

Urine was divided into unconjugated and glucuronide- and sulfate-conjugated fractions subjected to paper, thin-layer, and liquid chromatography, and to various group reactions (ultraviolet absorption, blue tetrazolium reduction, and the Porter-Silber, Zimmerman and Pettinkoffer tests). In some instances, binding to corticosteroid-binding globulin or to low-specificity steroid antibodies was used to screen for the presence of steroids in urinary extracts. No abnormality was detected by these procedures. In addition, the specific determination of the tetrahydro derivatives of the following steroids gave subnormal levels: aldosterone, cortisol, cortisone, corticosterone, 18-hydroxy-11-deoxycorticosterone, and 18-hydroxy-compound A. Although these procedures failed to reveal an abnormality, the possibility remained that an unpredicted steroid structure was being missed. Unfortunately, there is no general analytic reaction for steroids. Therefore, the next approach was to screen urinary extracts for an unknown substance solely on the basis of mass.

165

This was done first with the flame ionization detector of the gas chromatograph and then with the total ion monitor of the mass spectrometer to detect substances in the gas chromatographic effluent. With the latter technique, it was possible to detect several urinary steroids that were not revealed by less sensitive procedures, but the pattern was normal.

Analysis of Plasma

Plasma extracts exhibited subnormal levels of aldosterone, corticosterone, and 11-deoxycorticosterone, and in addition, G. Abraham (*unpublished observations*) found subnormal levels of pregnenolone, progesterone, and their 17-hydroxy derivatives.

Bioassay

The negative results obtained by chemical analysis suggested that if an abnormal steroid was present, its level was too low to be detected. A parallel investigation was therefore undertaken in which plasma and urinary extracts were screened for mineralocorticoid activity in search of active fractions that could be identified and purified for subsequent chemical analysis. These efforts, undertaken with the help of other investigators, are summarized in Table 1. An experiment directed to the question of enhanced sensitivity of the patient's tissues to steroids was included and gave normal results.

Table 1 shows that only the urinary fraction of steroid conjugates liberated by sulfatase or solvolysis was found to have mineralocorticoid activity by J. Sennett (*unpublished observations*). Activity persisted in some instances after chromatographic subfractionation on LH 20 columns. Gas chromatographic/ mass spectroscopic analysis of these fractions did not reveal the presence of steroids, although the amounts may have been below the limit of sensitivity. Efforts to confirm the presence of mineralocorticoid activity in the steroid sulfate fraction in two other laboratories were unsuccessful.

PATTERN OF PERIPHERAL STEROID METABOLISM

The preceding studies appeared to exclude a high steroid output syndrome, but did not exclude a more subtle abnormality in which a steroid was formed that was more active than either or both of the two normal final hormonal products, aldosterone and cortisol. Such a product might be secreted by the adrenal or, alternatively, formed by peripheral metabolism of a normal secretory product as, for example, in the conversion of testosterone to its 5α-dihydro derivative (2). This latter possibility was evaluated by studying the fate of administered tracer steroid hormones. As shown in Table 2, the overall pattern of metabolism of aldosterone was normal, including the formation of the pH 1 conjugate. A striking abnormality, however, was the large fraction of

TABLE 1. *Search for a biologically active factor in a juvenile syndrome of hypertensive hypokalemic alkalosis (patient L. K.)*

Assay	Investigator[a]	Activity[b]
Plasma		
Mineralocorticoid receptor binding	J. D. Baxter San Francisco, CA	−
Urinary extracts		
Free fraction		
Toad urinary bladder	D. Marver and I. S. Edelman San Francisco, CA	−
Sheep parotid Na/K	D. A. Denton et al. Melbourne, Australia	−
Adrenalectomized rat	J. A. Sennett and G. W. Liddle Nashville, TN	−
Glucuronide fraction		
Adrenalectomized rat	J. A. Sennett and G. W. Liddle Nashville, TN	−
Sulfate fraction		
Adrenalectomized rat	J. A. Sennett and G. W. Liddle Nashville, TN	+
	J. W. Funder et al. Melbourne, Australia	−
	R. D. Brown Rochester, MN	−
Lymphocyte		
Sensitivity to glucocorticoids (inhibition of phytohemagglutinin blast transformation)	P. F. Palmberg St. Louis, MO	−

[a]Unpublished observations.
[b]+, Activity increased; − activity not increased.

cortisol (averaging 43%) that was excreted in unconjugated form, compared to a normal value of less than 5%. The metabolism of compound S showed the same striking abnormality of marked increase in the fraction of unconjugated urinary metabolites. The percentage of corticosterone metabolites in the unconjugated fraction may have been slightly increased, but the abnormality

TABLE 2. *Steroid metabolism in a juvenile syndrome of hypertensive hypokalemic alkalosis (patient L. K.)*

Steroid	Urinary fraction %	
	Unconjugated	Glucuronide
Aldosterone[a]	2.5	30
Cortisol	43	12
Corticosterone	8.0	21
Compound S	55	20

[a]pH 1 conjugate (18-glucuronide) accounted for 11.5%.

was not as striking as it was in the case of cortisol and compound S. Thus, it appeared that this defect in metabolism involved largely those corticosteroids having the 17α-hydroxy group in their side chain.

COMPOSITION OF THE UNCONJUGATED (FREE) FRACTION

The marked increase in the percentage excretion of unconjugated metabolites could have been caused by a defect in the step involving conjugation with glucuronic acid. This possibility was evaluated by examining the steroidal components of the labeled unconjugated fraction of urine by means of reverse (carrier) isotope dilution. If impaired glucuronidation was the mechanism, then the unconjugated fraction should be composed largely of the normal tetrahydro metabolites of cortisol. Table 3 shows, however, that tetrahydrocortisol and tetrahydrocortisone together accounted for only a small part (15%) of the unconjugated fraction. Larger amounts of these steroids, detected by gas chromatography/mass spectrometry, were present in the glucuronide fraction. Thus, the defect involved incomplete reduction of cortisol to tetrahydro derivatives rather than impaired glucuronidation of the tetrahydro form. In addition, the defective formation of the tetrahydro derivatives of cortisol was relative rather than absolute.

Since cortisol secretion in this patient was very low under base-line conditions, the possiblity had to be considered that the abnormally high percentage excretion of unconjugated metabolites might be an adjustment to and a consequence of the low rate of cortisol secretion itself. The partition of conjugated and unconjugated Porter-Silber chromogenic steroids was therefore determined during a period of ACTH-stimulated cortisol secretion. When the glucuronide-conjugated fraction contained 5.8 mg of 17-hydroxy steroid metabolites, the unconjugated steroid fraction had an abnormally high content of 1.5 mg. Gas chromatographic/mass spectroscopic analysis of the ACTH-stimulated glucuronide fraction indicated the presence of normal tetrahydro and hexahydro metabolites of cortisol, such as tetrahydrocortisone, tetrahydrocortisol, and cortol.

TABLE 3. *Unconjugated urinary metabolites of cortisol in a juvenile syndrome of hypertensive hypokalemic alkalosis (patient L. K.)*

Steroid	Percent of unconjugated fraction
Cortisol	16.7
4,5-Dihydrocortisol	27.3
20-Dihydrocortisol	32.3
Tetrahydrocortisol	11.9
Tetrahydrocortisone	2.7

Table 3 shows that the normally predominant component of this unconjugated urinary fraction, cortisol, accounted for only 16.7%. The striking abnormality was that more than half of the unconjugated steroid fraction was
composed of dihydro derivatives formed by reducing either the C-20 ketone or
the 4,5 double bond. These dihydro metabolites of cortisol were quantitated
by the addition of carrier 20β-dihydrocortisol and 5α-dihydrocortisol. The
specific stereochemical assignments, however, cannot yet be regarded as
definitive. The separation techniques of paper and thin-layer chromatography
that were used separated the 20α- and 20β-forms, but the separation of the 5α-
and 5β-epimers proved to be more difficult. Although the latter were well
separated by gas chromatography of the methoxime trimethylsilyl ether derivatives, using OV-101 as stationary phase, 5α-dihydrocortisol had the same
retention time as cortisol. When this gas chromatographic technique was
applied to the patient's urinary extract, we did not detect any 5β-dihydrocorti-
sol. Since the presence of one of the 5-dihydro epimers had already been
demonstrated by reverse isotope dilution and conventional chromatography,
which readily separated cortisol from its 5α-dihydro derivatives, there was
indirect evidence for the presence predominantly of the 5α-form. For the more
definitive detection and quantitation of the 5α-dihydro derivative, two independent methods currently being developed appear to be promising. One
utilizes a high pressure, high performance liquid chromatogram column in
which all relevant metabolites are well separated. Another makes use of
capillary column–gas chromatography/mass spectrometry together with selective monitoring of specific ions.

RELATIONSHIP OF METABOLIC ABNORMALITY TO CLINICAL SYNDROME

Cortisol normally accounts for 90% of the unconjugated fraction, but little
information is available on the normal rates of excretion of dihydro metabolites of this fraction. The mean excretion of urinary free cortisol in this patient
in four base-line specimens was 8.6 ± 2.3 SD μg/day and is subnormal in
relation to the normal adult mean of 33 to 56 μg/day (3,4). Since the patient's
excretion of the 4,5 dihydro metabolite was almost twice that of cortisol, the
estimated excretion of the dihydro form would be approximately 15 μg/day.
Marver and Edelman (5) have obtained the following evidence to indicate that
5α-dihydrocortisol is a potential mineralocorticoid: (a) it promotes sodium
transport in the isolated toad urinary bladder; (b) it binds with a relatively high
affinity to the aldosterone receptors of rat kidney; and (c) it shows less binding
to corticosteroid-binding globulin than cortisol, so that a given plasma concentration is potentially more effective. It is not yet certain, however, whether
patient L. K. produces sufficient amounts of 5α-dihydrocortisol to account for
her syndrome of mineralocorticoid excess. In addition, as cited above, the
stereochemistry of the urinary dihydro metabolite has not yet been rigorously

established. If the predominant presence of the 5α-dihydro isomer can be confirmed by independent analytic methods, this itself would represent a clear abnormality because 5β-metabolites normally predominate in man.

Although a relationship between the observed abnormality in cortisol metabolism and the patient's syndrome of mineralocorticoid excess has not yet been established, it would seem unlikely that the two phenomena are entirely unrelated. In any case, the possible biological activity of 5α-reduced metabolites in a patient with a defect leading to the accumulation of such metabolites appears to be a promising avenue for further investigation in this and other hypertensive patients.

SUMMARY

A juvenile syndrome of hypertensive hypokalemic alkalosis, associated with subnormal production of known corticosteroids, was subjected to an exhaustive search for overproduction of an unknown steroid factor. The only steroid abnormality detected was a relative defect in the reduction of Ring A to form tetrahydro metabolites, particularly for steroids with the 17α-hydroxy-corticosteroid side chain. This resulted in the accumulation and increased urinary excretion of partially reduced dihydro forms whose mineralocorticoid activity may be an etiologic factor in the hypertensive syndrome.

ACKNOWLEDGMENTS

This work was supported by the Veterans Administration and NIH Grant No. AM 14040-08.

REFERENCES

1. New, M. I., and Levine, L. S. (1977): An unidentified ACTH-stimulable adrenal steroid in childhood hypertension, *this volume*.
2. Bruchovsky, N., and Wilson, J. D. (1968): The conversion of testosterone to 5α-androstan-17β-ol-3-one by rat prostate *in vivo* and *in vitro*. *J. Biol. Chem.*, 243:2012–2021.
3. Murphy, B. E. P. (1968): Clinical evaluation of urinary cortisol determinations by competitive protein-binding radioassay. *J. Clin. Endocrinol. Metab.*, 28:343–348.
4. Hsu, T. H., and Bledsoe, T. (1970): Measurement of urinary free corticoids by competitive protein-binding radioassay in hypoadrenal states. *J. Clin. Endocrinol. Metab.*, 30:443–448.
5. Marver, D., and Edelman, I. S., *personal communication*.

Juvenile Hypertension, edited by
M. I. New and L. S. Levine. Raven
Press, New York © 1977.

Plasma Deoxycorticosterone Concentrations in the Adrenal Enzymatic Deficiencies Causing Hypertension

Edward G. Biglieri

*Medical Service, San Francisco General Hospital, and the Department of Medicine,
University of California, San Francisco, California 94110*

The endogenous plasma concentration of deoxycorticosterone (DOC) that must be achieved to effect increases in blood pressure, potassium depletion, and suppression of plasma renin activity (PRA) is not well defined (1). The critical concentration is particularly difficult to establish when other steroids are present in normal or increased amounts and when the mineralocorticoid hormone (MCH) potency equals or exceeds that of DOC. This is invariably true in patients with adrenal malignancies, ectopic adrenocorticotropin (ACTH)-producing neoplasms, or aldosterone-producing adenomas, and is occasionally true in patients with Cushing's syndrome or disease (2,3). Patients with congenital adrenal hyperplasia with hypertension, the 11β-hydroxylation deficiency syndrome (11-OHDS), and the 17α-hydroxylation deficiency syndrome (17-OHDS) provide a unique opportunity to examine the effect of elevated levels of their principal mineralocorticoid hormone DOC in the presence of limited amounts of other adrenal steroids (4–6).

MATERIALS AND METHODS

Seven patients with the 17-OHDS ranged in age from 15 to 36 years and had the biochemical findings of reduced cortisol and aldosterone and increased DOC and corticosterone production, suppressed PRA, blood pressures ranging from 140/100 to 220/140 mm Hg, and hypokalemia ranging from 2.3 to 2.8 meq/liter. These cases are summarized elsewhere (7). A single female patient with the 11-OHDS became virilized at 15 years of age and had elevated urinary levels of pregnanetriol, 17-ketosteroids, and tetrahydro-11-deoxycortisol, elevated secretory rate of DOC, and reduced production of aldosterone and cortisol.

171

Secretory rates of DOC were measured and quantitated by the technique described for this laboratory after intravenous injection of 3 μCi of DOC-1-2-^{3}H (5). Plasma DOC concentrations were measured by radioimmunoassay. Separation and isolation of the DOC derivative deoxycorticosterone acetate (DOCA) was achieved by paper chromatography. Quantitation of the DOCA was accomplished by using antibodies generated to DOC-hemisuccinate coupled to rabbit gamma-globulin. The normal range of DOC (10 subjects) at 8 a.m. after overnight recumbency was 4 to 14 ng/dl.

Derived plasma DOC concentrations for the patients reported herein and for those in the literature were calculated from secretory rate data only, using the mean metabolic clearance rate (MCR) for DOC of 1,100 liters/24 hr, which was obtained in two patients with 17-OHDS in this laboratory by a constant infusion technique (8). This value is similar to the DOC MCR (956 ± 69 liters/ 24 hr) obtained in three normal subjects by the single injection and constant infusion techniques (9) and other reports of a DOC MCR range of 750 to 1,600 liters/24 hr (10,11). Written consent was obtained after patients were informed of the investigational nature of these studies, which were approved by the University of California, San Francisco, Committee on Human Research.

Results

Measured Plasma DOC Concentrations. DOC levels were considerably elevated in four patients with the 17-OHDS (Table 1). The mean value was 315.2 ng/dl, and the range was 172.5 to 484.0 ng/dl.

Derived Plasma DOC Concentrations. In seven patients with the 17-OHDS, the mean secretory rate of DOC was 2,873 ± 705 μg/24 hr, and the range was 1,400 to 5,100 μg/24 hr (Table 2). The derived plasma DOC concentrations using the MCR of two patients with this disorder were remarkably similar to the 8 a.m. values obtained by direct measurement. The mean value was 260.6 ± 60.6 ng/dl. The secretory rate of DOC in the patient with 11-OHDS was 6,600 μg/24 hr, and the derived plasma DOC level was 600 ng/dl.

Circadian Rhythm of Plasma DOC in 17-OHDS. In two patients, a nadir

TABLE 1. Measured plasma DOC at 8 a.m. in patients with 17-OHDS

Patient no.	Plasma DOC (ng/dl)
1	172.5
2	370.6
3	484.0
4	233.3
Mean	315.2
Normal range	4–14

TABLE 2. *Derived plasma DOC from secretory rate in patients with 17- and 11-OHDS*

Patient no.	DOC secretory rate (μg/24 hr)	Derived plasma DOC (ng/dl)
17-OHDS		
1	1,925	172.5
2	2,344	213.1
3	5,100	464.0
5	1,400	125.6
6	5,019	456.3
7	1,453	132.1
Mean	2,873 ± 705	260.6 ± 60.6
11-OHDS		
1	6,600	600.0
Normal range	50–350	—

occurred between 8 and 12 p.m. and the peak level between 4 and 8 a.m. Samples were obtained every 4 hr.

DISCUSSION

The elevations observed in both measured and derived plasma DOC concentrations are quite similar. The magnitude of the increase is probably essential for the development of increased blood pressure, potassium depletion, and sodium retention, which are invariably present in patients with 17-OHDS and are often observed in those with 11-OHDS. It is of considerable interest that from MCH receptor assay techniques (12) we can predict that a value of plasma DOC concentration 100 ng/dl or greater would effect inhibition of the binding of aldosterone and bring about a significant MCH response. The levels observed in these studies also compare favorably with the derived plasma DOC levels (based on secretory rates only) in other reports of these disorders (4,6,13–15) (Table 3). Mean DOC levels of 698.2 and 669.2 ng/dl were calculated in the 17- and 11-OHDS patients, respectively. After 3 consecutive days of intramuscular injection of 10 mg DOCA every 12 hr, an 8 a.m. level of DOC of 980 ng/dl was achieved (16), using the DOC radioimmunoassay described.

A circadian rhythm for DOC is present in patients with congenital adrenal hyperplasia that is similar to rhythms described for other ACTH-dependent steroids (17) and forms the rationale for therapeutic management with small doses of glucocorticoid hormones at night. This is relevant to patients with 17-OHDS who usually have exquisite sensitivity to such hormones (7).

Continued administration of DOCA to normal subjects does not result in hypertension. Chronic and quantitatively similar elevations of DOC concentrations in patients with 17-OHDS and 11-OHDS do not consistently produce

TABLE 3. *Derived plasma DOC from secretory rates reported in the literature*

DOC secretory rate (μg/24 hr)	Derived plasma DOC (ng/dl)	Reference no.
17-OHDS		
760	69.1	14
3,700	116.4	13
21,000	1,909.1	15
Mean 8,486	698.2	—
11-OHDS		
22,980	2,089.1	6
5,910	537.2	6
5,310	282.7	6
4,170	379.1	6
2,000	181.8	4
6,000	545.4	4
Mean 7,728	669.2	—

increases in blood pressure and alter electrolyte metabolism. These elevations occur when cortisol and aldosterone production are diminished or absent. However, other steroids may modify these results. The increased DOC levels in patients with 17-OHDS are accompanied by concentrations of corticosterone comparable to and often greater than normal cortisol levels. Similarly, in patients with 11-OHDS, the concurrent steroid in high concentrations is 11-deoxycortisol (6,7). Both corticosterone and 11-deoxycortisol, by virtue of their greater concentrations and affinities for corticosteroid-binding globulin, will make more "free" DOC and the MCH of consequence available in patients with these reduced aldosterone production states (Fig. 1).

Increased blood pressure and hypokalemia are always present in patients with 17-OHDS. The lack of a similar consistency in patients with 11-OHDS could be related to the anti-MCH renal effects of 17-hydroxyprogesterone (18), which is always elevated in patients with 17-OHDS. Progesterone, although not invariably elevated, could also contribute to a similar effect, depending on the degree of the enzyme deficiency (19).

ACKNOWLEDGMENTS

This study was supported in part by U.S. Public Health Service Research Grants HE-11046 from the National Heart Institute and AM-06415 from the National Institute of Arthritis and Metabolic Diseases. The studies were carried out in the General Clinical Research Center (RR-00083) at San Francisco General Hospital, with support by the Division of Research Resources, National Institutes of Health.

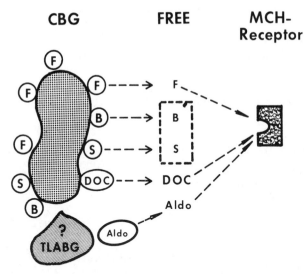

FIG. 1. Hypothetic importance of other steroids on availability of DOC and aldosterone (Aldo) to MCH receptor [TLABG, transcortin-like aldosterone-binding globulin (15)]. Increased amounts of corticosterone (B) and 11-deoxycortisol (S) in absence of cortisol (F) would make DOC more accessible to MCH receptor.

REFERENCES

1. Brown, J. J., Ferriss, J. B., Fraser, R., Lever, A. F., Love, D. R., Robertson, J. I. S., and Wilson, A. (1972): Apparently isolated excess deoxycorticosterone in hypertension. *Lancet,* 2:243–247.
2. Biglieri, E. G., Slaton, P. E., Jr., Schambelan, M., and Kronfield, S. J. (1968): Hypermineralocorticoidism. *Am. J. Med.,* 45:170–175.
3. Schambelan, M., Slaton, P. E., Jr., and Biglieri, E. G. (1971): Mineralocorticoid production in hyperadrenocorticism: Role in pathogenesis of hypokalemic alkalosis. *Am. J. Med.,* 51:299–303.
4. New, M. I., and Seaman, M. P. (1970): Secretion rates of cortisol and aldosterone precursors in various forms of congenital adrenal hyperplasia. *J. Clin. Endocrinol. Metab.,* 30:361.
5. Biglieri, E. G., Herron, M. A., and Brust, N. (1966): 17-Hydroxylation deficiency in man. *J. Clin. Invest.,* 45:1946–1954.
6. Loras, B., Roux, H., Dazord, A., and Bertrand, J. (1969): A study of the variations in the secretion rates of cortisol, corticosterone, aldosterone and deoxycorticosterone in four cases of congenital adrenal hyperplasia due to deficiency of 11β-hydroxylase. In: *Progress in Endocrinology,* edited by C. Gual and F. J. G. Ebling, pp. 1149–1159. Excerpta Medica Foundation, Amsterdam.
7. Biglieri, E. G. (1977): Adrenal enzymatic defects in hypertension. In: *Hypertension,* edited by J. Genest. McGraw-Hill, New York, *in press.*
8. Tait, J. F., Little, B., Tait, S. A. S., and Flood, C. (1962): The metabolic clearance rate of aldosterone in pregnant and nonpregnant subjects estimated by both single-injection and constant-infusion methods. *J. Clin. Invest.,* 41:2093–2100.
9. Schambelan, M., and Biglieri, E. G. (1972): Deoxycorticosterone production and regulation in man. *J. Clin. Endocrinol. Metab.,* 34:695–703.
10. Messerli, F. H., Nowaczynski, W., Honda, M., and Genest, J. (1975): Effects of ACTH and angiotensin II in steroid metabolism. In: *Program of the Fifty-Seventh Annual Meeting of the Endocrine Society,* p. 61.

11. Nolten, W., Vecsei, P., Köhler, M., Purjesz, I., and Wolff, H. P. (1968): Untersuchungen über Sekretion und Stoffwechsel von Desoxycorticosteron an Gesunden und Kranken. *Verh. Dtsch. Ges. Inn. Med.*, 74:1218–1221.
12. Baxter, J. D., Matulich, D. T., Spindler, B. J., Schambelan, M., Kawasaki, T. K., and Bartter, F. C. (1975): Aldosterone receptors and mineralocorticoid activity in hypertension. *Clin. Res.*, 23:386A.
13. Bricaire, H., Luton, J. P., Laudat, P., Legrand, J. C., Turpin, G., Corvol, P., and Lemmer, M. (1972): A new male pseudohermaphroditism associated with hypertension due to a block of 17α-hydroxylation. *J. Clin. Endocrinol. Metab.*, 35:67–72.
14. New, M. I. (1970): Male pseudohermaphroditism due to 17-alpha-hydroxylase defiency. *J. Clin. Invest.*, 49:1930–1941.
15. Nowaczynski, W., Kuchel, O., and Genest, J. (1975): Aldosterone, deoxycorticosterone, 18-hydroxydeoxycorticosterone and progesterone in benign essential hypertension. In: *Epidemiology and Control of Hypertension,* edited by O. Paul, pp. 265–296. Stratton Intercontinental Medical Book Corporation, New York.
16. Biglieri, E. G. (1976): *Unpublished observations.*
17. Fukushima, D. K., Finkelstein, J. W., Yoshida, K., Boyar, R. M., and Hellman, L. (1975): Pituitary-adrenal activity in untreated congenital adrenal hyperplasia. *J. Clin. Endocrinol. Metab.*, 40:1–12.
18. Jacobs, D. R., van der Poll, J., Gabrilove, J. L., and Soffer, L. J. (1961): 17α-Hydroxyprogesterone—a salt-losing steroid: Relation to congenital adrenal hyperplasia. *J. Clin. Endocrinol. Metab.*, 21:909–922.
19. Simopoulos, A. P., Marshall, J. R., Delea, C. S., and Bartter, F. C. (1975): Studies of the deficiency of 21-hydroxylation in patients with congenital adrenal hyperplasia. *J. Clin. Endocrinol. Metab.*, 32:438–443.

Juvenile Hypertension, edited by
M. I. New and L. S. Levine. Raven
Press, New York © 1977.

Steroid Receptors and Hypertension

Isidore S. Edelman

*Cardiovascular Research Institute, University of California School of Medicine,
San Francisco, California 94143*

There is a substantial body of evidence that all steroid hormones, including vitamin D, act in the following steps: The steroid enters the target cell from the blood (what the target cell sees, with the possible exception of the liver where there are fenestrated capillaries, is largely the free steroid, not the protein-bound steroid) and binds to the available receptor sites. If the steroid is an agonist, this results in the formation of an active complex that in turn binds to the chromosomal apparatus. The first measurable response is an increase in messenger RNA synthesis. In the case of aldosterone, the increase in synthesis of polyA(+)-RNA (putative mRNA) occurs in 15 to 30 min (1,2). After an hour, an increase in the synthesis of ribosomal RNA precursors becomes apparent (3). As a result of the increase in RNA synthesis, augmentation of protein synthesis ensues and produces some (perhaps all) of the physiological effects. In the isolated toad bladder, for example, we found a linear correlation between the magnitude of the increase in polyA(+)-RNA synthesis and that in sodium transport elicited by aldosterone (1,2).

Some of the properties of the aldosterone receptor in the mammalian kidney have been elucidated recently. In the adrenalectomized rat, ^{3}H-aldosterone was rapidly bound to the cytoplasmic form of the receptor, attaining a peak concentration in less than 2 min after intravenous injection (4).

The nuclear fraction that is purified by sedimentation through 2.2 M sucrose contains two binding components: Tris-soluble and KCl- (0.4 M) extractable forms. The appearance and disappearance of these two components are in parallel. During the first 10 min the quantity of ^{3}H-aldosterone–receptor complex in the cytoplasm falls continuously and that in the nucleus increases significantly, that is, almost a doubling of the nuclear content of the complex. Thereafter, there is a progressive fall in nuclear content of the complex but the nuclear:cytoplasmic ratio continues to increase. These results indicate the presence of a nuclear accumulation mechanism that depends on the binding of an active steroid to the cytoplasmic receptor.

Spirolactone also binds to the cytoplasmic receptor but does not generate the intranuclear form. Thus, spirolactone inhibits the action of aldosterone by denying access to the receptor site and forming a "dead" complex.

The fact that aldosterone is bound to the nucleus *in vivo* was indicated on autoradiographs of toad bladder epithelium based on dry-mount techniques in studies by Bogoroch (5). By grain counting, she found that ^{3}H-aldosterone was present in the nucleus at three times the abundance to that found in cytoplasm. In contrast, with an inactive steroid (e.g., ^{3}H-estradiol-17β), the distribution between cytoplasm and nucleus was random.

To demonstrate that the intranuclear binding system for aldosterone is derived from the cytoplasm, Marver and I (4) made use of a reconstitution system. ^{3}H-aldosterone was added to preformed rat kidney cytosol and then mixed with "naive" nuclei. The intranuclear forms appeared as the cytoplasmic steroid–receptor complex disappeared, implying transfer to the nucleus. Moreover, the ^{3}H-aldosterone complexes in both cytoplasm and nucleus have identical steroid specificities, including stereoisomeric requirements (e.g., 17α-isoaldosterone does not bind to either form and has no action on Na$^+$ transport).

From cross-competition experiments, it is now clear that the receptors do not have absolute specificity for the primary steroid ligand. Thus, aldosterone, if present in high enough concentrations, will occupy glucocorticoid receptor sites and vice versa. Illicit occupancy may account for many previously mysterious phenomena, such as aldosterone-induced steroid diabetes, salt retention evoked by glucocorticoids, or sex steroids.

There are now emerging generalizations from recent information on steroid receptors: (a) Failure to occupy the receptor implies no action via that pathway. (b) Occupancy implies either an agonist effect, an antagonist effect, or both. (c) If a steroid is a partial agonist, and occupies all of the receptor sites, the sum of the agonist and antagonist effects should add up to a 100% action, as compared to a pure agonist. The latter prediction has been clearly demonstrated for 11-deoxycortisol in the toad bladder system where it possesses a 30% agonist and 70% antagonist effect as compared to aldosterone. Similar results have been obtained with a series of glucocorticoids by Samuels and Tomkins (6).

One of the intriguing insights that is coming into focus is that the receptor dictates the biological response. Thus, in the liver, glucocorticoids augment gluconeogenesis. If a steroid other than a glucocorticoid (e.g., progesterone) occupies the glucocorticoid receptor site, it can either mimic the action of the glucocorticoid (i.e., stimulate gluconeogenesis) or inhibit the action of an authentic glucocorticoid, but does not have the option of dictating an entirely new response. In the experiments of Samuels and Tomkins (6), progesterone was a partial agonist and partial antagonist in inducing tyrosine aminotransferase, a glucocorticoid-induced enzyme.

An important point to bear in mind is that the effectiveness of any one steroid will be strongly influenced by the degree of occupancy of the receptor by other steroids. Thus, in New and Levine's studies (7) on the hypertensive child, the apparent ineffectiveness of aldosterone may simply reflect prior occupancy of the aldosterone receptor by an as yet unidentified steroid.

Another point of interest is that a single steroid present in excess would be expected to occupy both its own receptor (licit) and any other receptors that fall within the range of its dissociation constant (illicit). In the case presented by New and Levine (7), the unidentified steroid (presumed) appears to function both as a glucocorticoid and as a mineralocorticoid; plasma cortisol and aldosterone concentrations are low, ACTH is suppressed, and the patient bears all of the stigmata of a mineralocorticoid type of hypertension. Since the patient does not have the clinical manifestations of either hyper- or hypoglucocorticoidism, one inference to be drawn is that steroid x has titrated all of the mineralocorticoid receptor sites but only part of the glucocorticoid sites, which is sufficient to suppress plasma ACTH levels but not enough to produce a Cushing's syndrome.

The failure to detect a corticosteroid in abundance, by either gas-liquid chromatography or mass spectrometry, raises the possibility of an abnormality other than an abnormal steroid. In theory, a mineralocorticoid-excess state could result either from abnormal receptors (one that is exquisitely sensitive to low concentrations of aldosterone) or from constitutive rather than inducible gene sites. The latter possibility is essentially ruled out by the response to spirolactone in the child described by New and Levine (7). The former is also unlikely for two reasons: (a) There is no precedent for genetically determined "superreceptors;" and (b) this would not explain the low-plasma cortisol and ACTH levels.

ACKNOWLEDGMENT

This work was supported by U.S.P.H.S. Program Project Grant No. HL-06285.

REFERENCES

1. Rossier, B. C., Wilce, P. A., and Edelman, I. S. (1974): Kinetics of RNA labeling in toad bladder epithelium: Effects of aldosterone and related steroids. *Proc. Natl. Acad. Sci. USA,* 71:3101–3105.
2. Wilce, P. A., Rossier, B. C., and Edelman, I. S. (1976): Actions of aldosterone on poly (A)(+)-RNA and Na$^+$ transport in the toad bladder. *Biochemistry,* 15:4279–4285.
3. Wilce, P. A., Rossier, B. C., and Edelman, I. S. (1976): Actions of aldosterone on rRNA and Na$^+$ transport in the toad bladder. *Biochemistry,* 15:4286–4292.
4. Marver, D., Goodman, D., and Edelman, I. S. (1972): Relationships between renal cytoplasmic and nuclear aldosterone receptors. *Kidney Int.,* 1:210–223.
5. Bogoroch, R., cited in, Edelman, I. S. (1973): Regulation of transepithelial sodium transport by aldosterone. In: *Transport Mechanisms in Epithelia,* p. 185. Munksgaard, Copenhagen.
6. Samuels, H. H., and Tomkins, G. M. (1970): Relation of steroid structure to enzyme induction in hepatoma tissue culture cells. *J. Mol. Biol.,* 52:57–74.
7. New, M., and Levine, L. S. (1977): An unidentified ACTH-stimulable adrenal steroid in childhood hypertension, *this volume.*

Juvenile Hypertension, edited by
M. I. New and L. S. Levine. Raven
Press, New York © 1977.

Hemodynamic Abnormalities of Adolescent Hypertension

Harriet P. Dustan and Robert C. Tarazi

*Research Division, The Cleveland Clinic Foundation, The Cleveland Clinic
Educational Foundation, Cleveland, Ohio 44106*

The early studies of the hemodynamics of hypertension showed cardiac output to be normal and peripheral resistance to be elevated. Thus, for years the belief was strongly held that the only important abnormality of hypertension was an increased resistance which reflected vasoconstriction. Perhaps, as a corollary, it was also believed that diastolic hypertension was the important type, whereas elevation of systolic pressure was considered relatively unimportant. The last 15 years have brought a great change in our knowledge of the hemodynamics of hypertension. Now we know there is a broad spectrum of abnormalities of both cardiac output and vascular resistance. In any etiologic type, output may be high, normal, or low (1–7). Resistance is usually elevated but often when output is elevated, it may be normal. In that circumstance, arterial pressure is elevated because resistance has failed to adjust downward in response to increased flow, as occurs normally. In addition to the recognition of the hemodynamic heterogeneity of hypertension, there is a growing acceptance of the fact that systolic hypertension represents abnormalities of arterial pressure regulation, just as does diastolic hypertension, and is an important determinant of vascular complications (8,9).

Many factors control arterial blood pressure. Those that determine it directly are flow and resistance (as expressed by the formula MAP = CO × TPR, where mean arterial pressure = cardiac output × total peripheral resistance), aortic impedance, and diastolic arterial volume. The indirect determinants influence the direct determinants; these are autonomic neural activity, extracellular fluid volumes, electrolyte-active steroids, and the renal pressor system.

Whereas information concerning abnormalities of arterial pressure control has come from studies of animal models of hypertension and hypertensive adults, it is known that hypertension in young people is often labile and

181

characterized by modest elevations of CO, with a normal or slightly increased vascular resistance (10,11). This finding raises the question of whether all hypertension begins with increased systemic flow (12) and necessitates a hemodynamic survey of hypertension in adolescents to determine whether increased CO is the hemodynamic hallmark, regardless of the etiology of raised pressure.

This report describes findings in a group of adolescents and young adults with hypertension of varying etiology.[1] The results show that in this age group there is the same hemodynamic heterogeneity that has been found in adult hypertensives.

METHODS OF STUDY

Patients Studied

The patients studied were 55 young people ranging in age from 12 to 25 years. Forty-three (38 males, 5 females) were considered to have idiopathic hypertension because extensive investigations had failed to show any of the known causes. For the rest of the patients, five had aortic coarctation, two had renal arterial stenosis, three had renal parenchymal disease, and two had Cushing's syndrome. The relatively large numbers of patients with idiopathic hypertension do not, of course, reflect the true occurrence of this type in young people but merely represent the class of patients referred for hemodynamic studies. Because clinical studies had failed to show any of the known causes of hypertension, the patients were referred because of the possibility that elevated pressure was caused by a high CO. The fact that there were so many males in this group reflects the concern generated by the finding of hypertension in boys and young men on examination to determine their eligibility for competitive sports.

Hemodynamic Studies

Hemodynamic studies were performed in the morning after an overnight fast and without sedation (13). The procedure was carefully explained to the patients the day before and consent obtained from them and their parents, when appropriate. Arterial pressure was continuously recorded from a catheter introduced percutaneously into the brachial artery and advanced to the axillary artery or aorta. CO was determined in replicate, using indocyanine green, and expressed as cardiac index (liters/min/m²). TPR was calculated from MAP and cardiac index, and expressed in arbitrary U/m². Heart rate (HR) was counted from a continuously recorded electrocardiogram. The results

---

[1]These data formed the basis for a previous report (*Pediatric Nephrology*, Vol. II, edited by J. Strauss, Stratton Intercontinental Medical Book Corp., New York, 1976, pp. 385–392).

TABLE 1. *Hemodynamic functions as measured in 29 normotensive control subjects (mean age 35 years)*

Hemodynamic function	Mean	SEM
MAP	89 mm Hg	± 1.8
PP	51 mm Hg	± 1.3
HR	67 beats/min	± 1.7
CI	3.1 liters/min/m²	± 0.08
TPR	29 U/m²	± 0.83

MAP, mean arterial pressure; PP, pulse pressure; HR, heart rate; CI, cardiac index; TPR, total peripheral resistance.

obtained were compared with the normal values of these functions from our laboratory, which are given in Table 1. However, the 29 normotensive controls were older (mean age 35 years) than the young people studied. Because of the likely possibility that if we had the opportunity to examine normotensive people of the same age group, we would have found slightly higher values for cardiac index than were found in the older individuals, the results of this study in the adolescents were not subjected to statistical analysis.

RESULTS

Idiopathic Hypertension

The results of idiopathic hypertension are shown in Table 2. Although all 43 patients had been diagnosed as having hypertension because of pressures equal to or greater than 140/90 at three or more readings, in 32 patients arterial pressure was equal to or less than 130/80 during hemodynamic studies. It seemed therefore advisable to analyze the results according to the pressure at the time of the study. The group with higher pressure, compared to that with lower pressure, had higher cardiac index (3.6 versus 3.0 liters/min/m²), faster HR (80 versus 74 beats/min), wider pulse pressure (60 versus 50 mm Hg), and

TABLE 2. *Hemodynamic functions[a] in 43 young "essential" hypertensives aged 12 to 25 years*

BP at time of study	≤ 130/80	> 130/80
Number	32	11
MAP	95	110
PP	50	60
HR	74	80
CI	3.0	3.6
TPR	30	31

[a]Units for hemodynamic variables are given as in Table 1.

TABLE 3. *Distribution of cardiac index in 43 young "essential" hypertensives and 29 normotensive control subjects*

Subjects	Cardiac index (liters/min/m²)		
	< 2.7	2.7 to 3.3	>3.3
Hypertensives			
Number	4	11	28
Percent	9	26	65
Normotensives			
Number	6	16	7
Percent	20	55	25

the same TPR (31 versus 30 U/m²). Although more than half of these patients had a CO higher than the upper limit of the normal range for our normal controls (Table 3), there were 15/43 who had normal or reduced CO.

Aortic Coarctation

Results in five patients (Table 4) show the variability of hemodynamic functions that characterizes any form of hypertension. Thus, hypertension was variably severe, pulse pressure ranged from normal to markedly elevated, HR from normal to elevated, cardiac index from normal to elevated, and TPR from normal to elevated.

Renovascular Hypertension

Two patients (Table 5) had nonatherosclerotic renal arterial stenosis causing hypertension. This type, at least in adults, is often characterized by slightly elevated CO. In the 2 patients studied, the results were remarkably similar and therefore the values were averaged. They show the same characteristics as those found in older people with renovascular hypertension (e.g., a slightly faster HR, an elevated cardiac index, and a slight elevation of vascular resistance). Surprisingly, for patients of this age, the pulse pressure was 76 mm Hg, which is distinctly abnormal.

TABLE 4. *Hemodynamic functions[a] in five patients with aortic coarctation*

Hemodynamic function	Mean value	Range
MAP	127	113–134
PP	74	45–93
HR	80	67–93
CI	3.5	2.8–4.3
TPR	37	31–47

[a]Units as given in Table 1.

TABLE 5. *Hemodynamic functions[a] in young patients with renal hypertension*

Hemodynamic function	Arterial stenosis[b]	Parenchymal disease		
		Patient no.		
		1	2	3
MAP	123	124	124	128
PP	76	82	63	73
HR	78	79	63	66
CI	3.8	4.8	3.2	3.0
TPR	33	26	38	48

[a]Units as given in Table 1.
[b]Values from the two patients were averaged because they were similar.

Renal Parenchymal Disease

When renal parenchymal disease was studied (Table 5), MAP was found to be the same for each patient, yet hemodynamic functions were distinctly different. In the first patient, cardiac index was markedly increased for a hypertensive and TPR was at the lower limit of the normal range. Thus, in this patient, high arterial pressure was an expression of the high CO, with failure of TPR to fall sufficiently to maintain normal pressure. In contrast, the other two patients had normal CO and elevated resistance; however, HR was normal in both. In all three, pulse pressure was elevated.

Cushing's Syndrome

The two women with Cushing's syndrome (Table 6) had markedly different arterial pressure levels during the hemodynamic study. In one, it was within the normal range and in the other, it was elevated. In the one with normal pressure, cardiac index was elevated and TPR, in response to this elevation, was reduced. In the other, with hypertension, cardiac index was below the normal range for adults and hypertension was maintained by a high vascular resistance.

TABLE 6. *Hemodynamic functions[a] in two young women with Cushing's syndrome*

Hemodynamic function	Patient	
	1	2
MAP	99	129
PP	73	56
HR	80	82
CI	4.0	2.4
TPR	25	53

[a]Units as given in Table 1.

DISCUSSION

One of the recurring features of hemodynamics of hypertension in adults has been the range of values found, even within the same etiologic group (1–7). This indicates individual variations in the factors determining high pressure, regardless of the initiating mechanisms. The results of studies in young people, as reported here, show the same variability. It has long been suggested that high CO initiates hypertension (14–16), and although our patients tended to have high flow, in some it was normal and in a few, even depressed. These results do not resolve the question concerning how hypertension begins, but they do show that low or normal CO can occur in relatively young hypertensives. If autoregulation had occurred and was responsible for maintaining pressure by increased vascular resistance (14–16), it must have occurred very early, as several of these patients had been known to be hypertensive for only a short time.

Lack of normal values of hemodynamic functions for this age group prohibits a statistical analysis of the frequency with which high systemic flow may characterize hypertension in young patients. It does not, however, detract from the data showing the broad spectrum of hemodynamics in all forms of hypertension.

The values obtained in idiopathic hypertension are similar to those reported previously in individuals somewhat older (1,10,11). They show that CO is well maintained—perhaps even elevated—while vascular resistance is normal. In the group that had arterial pressure greater than 130/80 at the examination, the higher pressure expressed a higher flow. This supports the concept that one of the important faults, even in the early phases of hypertension, is a failure of appropriate vasodilatation in response to increasing flow. In this regard, Lund-Johansen (11) has shown that young labile hypertensives differ in their hemodynamic responses to exercise from normotensives of similar age by a lesser fall in vascular resistance during exercise.

Generally speaking, aortic coarctation is associated with a wide pulse pressure and a slightly increased CO (17). The reason for the characteristic pressure seems easily explained by the diminished aortic capacity so that there is less surface area to absorb the kinetic energy of each systolic thrust (18). The average results for this group support that thesis because pulse pressure was increased as was also cardiac index. In this type of hypertension, as in all others, averaging the results obscured the heterogeneity of the findings. Thus, the slightly decreased pulse pressure found in one patient seemed noteworthy because it was associated with a cardiac index that was close to the lower limit of the normal range in adults, and this may be the reason why that patient had the lowest MAP of the entire group. In contrast, the patient with the highest pressure also had the widest pulse pressure and largest CO. It seems likely that in this form of hypertension, more than in all others, the correlation between pressure and flow would be a better one than that obtained in other forms of hypertension.

We have previously shown that hypertension in patients with renal arterial stenosis is often accompanied by slight increases in CO (5,6). The results obtained in these two younger patients showed also that hypertension was associated with both an elevated CO and an increased resistance. These findings probably reflect not only the peripheral vasoconstrictive action of angiotensin II but also its well-known stimulatory effects on the sympathetic nervous system (19,20).

The results for each patient with renal parenchymal disease were listed separately (Table 5) because of their marked differences. Fortuitously, MAP was practically identical for all three; in one instance, output was high and resistance was low, while in the other two, high pressure was an expression of high resistance. We had previously shown the same type of heterogeneity for hemodynamic functions in a larger group of patients with pyelonephritis (21). The very high CO found in one patient (no. 1) is reminiscent of the high-flow type of hypertension reported in patients with end-stage kidney disease (22). However, neither this patient nor the other two were azotemic, and because all three had normal hemoglobin, anemia cannot be the explanation.

The results in the two young women with Cushing's syndrome again show the same hemodynamic heterogeneity. Reasons for hypertension in Cushing's syndrome have not been provided by this or any other study. In contrast to the clear association of hypertension with positive salt and water balance that have been found for primary aldosteronism (23), these patients may have another factor; there is a growing body of evidence that in both animals and man there may be some steroid hypertensions that are not salt and water dependent (24,25).

SUMMARY

Previous studies of hemodynamic functions in hypertensive adults have failed to show consistent characteristics of flow and vascular resistance that depended on the etiologic type of hypertension. In spite of this, elevated CO has been suggested as the initiator of established hypertension in man as it seems to be in most experimental models. To investigate this possibility, we reviewed hemodynamic data available from a study of 55 young people ranging in age from 12 to 25 years (43 with idiopathic hypertension, 5 with aortic coarctation, 2 with renovascular hypertension, 3 with renal parenchymal disease, and 2 with Cushing's syndrome). The results show the same hemodynamic heterogeneity as that found in adult forms of hypertension, regardless of cause.

ACKNOWLEDGMENT

This study was supported in part by grant HL 6835 from the National Heart, Lung, and Blood Institute, National Institutes of Health, Bethesda, Maryland.

REFERENCES

1. Frohlich, E. D., Tarazi, R. C., and Dustan, H. P. (1969): Re-examination of the hemodynamics of hypertension. *Am. J. Med. Sci.,* 257:9.
2. Eich, R. H., Peters, R. J., Cuddy, R. P., Smulyan, H., and Lyons, R. H. (1962): The hemodynamics in labile hypertension. *Am. Heart. J.,* 63:188.
3. Bello, C. T., Sevy, R. W., and Harakal, C. (1965): Varying hemodynamic patterns in essential hypertension. *Am. J. Med. Sci.,* 250:58.
4. Finkielman, S., Worcel, M., and Agrest, A. (1965): Hemodynamic patterns in essential hypertension. *Circulation,* 31:356.
5. Frohlich, E. D., Ulrych, M., Tarazi, R. C., Dustan, H. P., and Page, I. H. (1967): A hemodynamic comparison of essential and renovascular hypertension. Cardiac output and total peripheral resistance, supine and tilted patients. *Circulation,* 35:289.
6. Frohlich, E. D., Ulrych, M., Tarazi, R. C., Dustan, H. P., and Page, I. H. (1968): Hemodynamics of renal arterial diseases and hypertension. *Am. J. Med. Sci.,* 255:29.
7. Tarazi, R. C., Ibrahim, M. M., Bravo. E. L., and Dustan, H. P. (1973): Hemodynamic characteristics of primary aldosteronism. *N. Engl. J. Med.,* 289:1330.
8. Stamler, J., Berkson, D. M., and Lindberg, H. A. (1972): Risk factors: Their role in the etiology and pathogenesis of the atherosclerotic diseases. In: *The Pathogenesis of Atherosclerosis,* edited by R. W. Wissler and J. C. Geer, p. 41. Williams & Wilkins, Baltimore, Md.
9. Kannel, W. B., Wolf, P. A., Verter, J., and McNamara, P. M. (1970): Epidemiologic assessment of the role of blood pressure in stroke. *JAMA,* 214:301.
10. Julius, S., and Conway, J. (1968): Hemodynamic studies in patients with borderline blood pressure elevation. *Circulation,* 38:282.
11. Lund-Johansen, P. (1967): Hemodynamic pattern in essential hypertension at rest and during muscular exercise. *Acta Med. Scand.,* 181(Suppl.):482.
12. Eich, R. H., Cuddy, R. P., and Smulyan, H. (1966): Hemodynamics in labile hypertension. A follow-up study. *Circulation,* 34:299.
13. Tarazi, R. C., and Dustan, H. P. (1972): Beta adrenergic blockade in hypertension. *Am. J. Cardiol.,* 29:633.
14. Borst, J. G. G. (1963): Hypertension explained by Starling's theory of circulation homeostasis. *Lancet,* 1:677.
15. Ledingham, J. M. (1971): Blood pressure regulation in renal failure. *J. R. Coll. Physicians, Lond.,* 5:103.
16. Guyton, A. C., and Coleman, T. G. (1969): Quantitative analysis of the pathophysiology of hypertension. *Circ. Res.,* 24 and 25(Suppl. I):1.
17. Culbertson, J. W., Eckstein, J. W., Kirkendall, W. M., and Bedell, G. (1957): General hemodynamics and splanchnic circulation in patients with coarctation of the aorta. *J. Clin. Invest.,* 36:1537.
18. Gupta, T. C., and Wiggers, C. J. (1970): Basic hemodynamic changes produced by aortic coarctation of different degrees. *Circulation,* 3:17.
19. Joy, M. D., and Lowe, R. D. (1970): The site of cardiovascular action of angiotensin II in the brain. *Clin. Sci.,* 39:327.
20. Khairallah, P. A., Davila, D., Papanicolaou, N., Glende, H. M., and Meyer, P. (1971): Effects of angiotensin infusion on catecholamine uptake and reactivity in blood vessels. *Circ. Res.,* 28 and 29(Suppl. II):96.
21. Frohlich, E. D., Tarazi, R. C., and Dustan, H. P. (1971): Hemodynamic and functional mechanisms in two renal hypertensions: Arterial and pyelonephritis. *Am. J. Med. Sci.,* 261:189.
22. Kim, K. E., Onesti, G., Schwartz, A. B., Chinitz, J. L., and Swartz, C. (1972): Hemodynamics of hypertension in chronic end-stage renal disease. *Circulation,* 46:456.
23. Bravo, E. L., Dustan, H. P., and Tarazi, R. C. (1973): Spironolactone as a nonspecific treatment for primary aldosteronism. *Circulation,* 48:491.
24. Scoggins, B. A., Coghlan, J. P., Cran, E. J., Denton, D. A., Fan, S. H., McDougall, J. G., Oddie, C. J., Robinson, P. M., and Shulkes, A. A. (1973): Experimental studies on the mechanism of adrenocorticotrophic hormone-induced hypertension in the sheep. *Clin. Sci. Mol. Med.,* 45(Suppl I):269.
25. New, M., and Ulick, S., (1976): New forms of childhood hypertension. In: *Conference on Childhood Hypertension,* March 26. Kroc Foundation, Santa Ynez Valley, California.

Juvenile Hypertension, edited by
M. I. New and L. S. Levine. Raven
Press, New York © 1977.

Hemodynamic Studies of Labile Essential Hypertension in Adolescents

*Andre Davignon, *Christian Rey, *,[1]Maurice Payot, †Pierre Biron, and **,†Jean-Guy Mongeau

*Department of Pediatrics, Services of *Cardiology and **Nephrology, Saint-Justine Hospital for Children, Montreal, Quebec H3T 1C5; and †Department of Pharmacology, University of Montreal, Montreal, Quebec H3C 3J7, Canada*

Although numerous hemodynamic studies have been devoted to labile essential hypertension, very few have included children and adolescents. Most researchers (3–6,12) have found a high cardiac index with normal or low peripheral resistance. Levy and co-workers (7) have found that peripheral resistance is elevated and cardiac index normal, but several reports from the United States (1) and France (10,11) favor the occurrence of both hemodynamic patterns.

Using echocardiography, we have studied 23 adolescents and young adults, age 6 to 23, suffering from labile essential hypertension. These patients were compared with 43 normotensive patients and 9 with renal hypertension.

Echocardiography is now a well-recognized noninvasive technique in studying anatomical heart malformations. Its value in studying the function of the left ventricle is, however, still subject to controversy.

Although this chapter is not the place to discuss in detail the value of echocardiography in studying the hemodynamics of hypertension, our colleagues in hemodynamics do believe it is indeed a reliable method for the following reasons:

(a) Feigenbaum and co-workers (2) have found an excellent correlation between the dimension of the left ventricle measured by echocardiography and by angiography.

(b) Lundstrom (8) has demonstrated a good reproducibility for the measurement of the left ventricular internal diameter by echocardiography.

(c) Eleven of our patients with essential labile hypertension were studied, at least, on two different occasions. In each case, the hemodynamic data

---

[1]*Present address:* Service of Cardiology, Albert Calvette Hospital, 59000 Lille, France.

represent the mean value of three readings. In 10 of 11 instances, the findings were almost identical.

The technique of echocardiography used in our center has been published in detail (9). In summary, after the patient was recumbent for half an hour, the blood pressure was determined by the Doppler ultrasonic technique. Simultaneously, a carotidogram was taken and mean blood pressure was determined by combining the reading obtained by the Doppler technique with planimetry of the carotidogram, using the Stefadouros technique.

Cardiac output was measured according to the formula:

$$CO = LVID\,(d)^3 - LVID\,(s)^3 \times HR$$

where CO = cardiac output; LVID = left ventricular internal diameter; and HR = heart rate. Heart rate was determined by averaging at least 10 RR intervals on the simultaneously taken electrocardiogram. Total peripheral resistance was calculated from the mean blood pressure and the cardiac output and expressed in μm/m^2.

Student's t-test was used to compare the mean values obtained in each hypertensive group with those of the normal group. A chi-square test was performed to evaluate the distribution of hyperkinetic versus hyperresistant patients.

The term "essential hypertension" was used for children with a blood pressure at rest over the 90th percentile for their age, on three different occasions, and with a normal intravenous pyelogram, blood chemistry, urinary vanillylmandelic acid, and renal function. On the day echocardiogram was performed, and after half an hour of rest, 11 of our 23 children with labile hypertension had "normal" blood pressure according to our previous definition; they were, however, hypertensive when compared to the group of normal children who were reported as the control group for echocardiography. Although such a fluctuation in blood pressure might bring difficulties in interpreting results, it was not a surprise to us, because, as shown in Fig. 1 from a preliminary study, the group of children with essential hypertension was more sensitive to anxiety and rest than other children.

RESULTS

Figure 2 shows the results of these hemodynamic studies on children with essential labile hypertension as compared to normal. It is apparent that the children with essential hypertension, as well as normal children, are divided approximately between hyperkinetics and hyperresistants.

In order to express these results in a more meaningful way, the term "index of kinetism" was used. The normal cardiac index averaged 4 liters/min/m^2 and the normal total peripheral resistance (TPR) 20 μm/m^2. The ratio CO/⅕TPR was used for the normal subjects. An index of kinetism over 1 reflects a hyperkinetic child and that below 1 reflects a hyperresistant child.

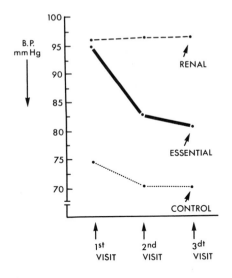

FIG. 1. Diastolic blood pressure of children taken at home on three consecutive visits. The group of children with essential hypertension shows a significant decrease between first and second visits, which is probably the result of anxiety, whereas normal or renal hypertensive patients do not show that difference.

Figure 3 shows the results of using such an index. Again, normal and essential hypertensive children are divided approximately and equally above and below the line of identity. The children with renal hypertension are all hyperresistants. In the group of essential hypertensives, 11 have an index over 1, and 14 below 1.

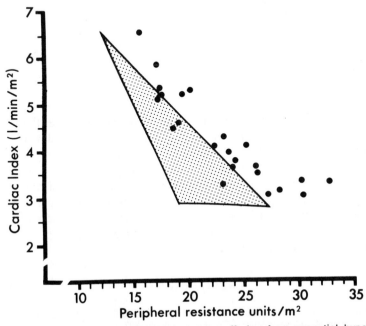

FIG. 2. Hemodynamic study of 23 adolescents suffering from essential hypertension. *Dotted area,* normal values; *filled circles,* hemodynamic status of one child.

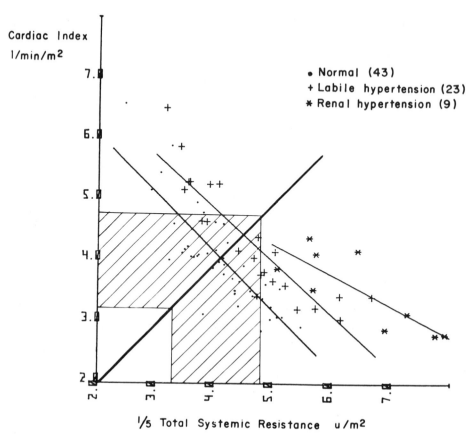

FIG. 3. Index of kinetism of adolescents. Children suffering from essential hypertension (+) are divided almost equally above and below the line of identity. *Shaded area,* 2 SD of normal values.

Hyperkinetic patients have a cardiac index significantly greater than normal ($p < 0.01$) and hyperresistant patients have an average peripheral resistance of 26.3 μm/m², which is again significantly higher than the normal ($p < 0.01$). Our results make improbable the hypothesis of Eich (1), whereby a young hypertensive person is first hyperkinetic and later becomes hyperresistant.

It is conceivable that essential labile hypertension may present itself, initially, as hyperkinetic or hyperresistant. In order to verify such a hypothesis, we are now in the process of studying hemodynamically the parents of our children with essential labile hypertension.

REFERENCES

1. Eich, R. H., Cuddy, R. P., Smulyan, H., and Lyons, R. H. (1966): Hemodynamics in labile hypertension. A follow-up study. *Circulation,* 34:299–307.

2. Feigenbaum, H., Popp, R. L., Wolfe, S. B., Troy, B. L., Pombro, J. F., Haine, C. L., and Dodge, H. T. (1972): Ultrasound measurements of the left ventricle. A correlative study with angiocardiography. *Arch. Intern. Med.,* 129:461–467.
3. Frohlich, E. D. (1973): Clinical significance of hemodynamic findings in hypertension. *Chest,* 64:94–99.
4. Hamer, J. (1968): Hemodynamics of hypertension. *Am. Heart J.,* 76:149–152.
5. Julius, S., Pascual, A. V., Sannerstedt, R., and Mitchell, C. (1971): Relationship between cardiac output and peripheral resistance in borderline hypertension. *Circulation,* 43:382–390.
6. Kuramoto, K., Murata, K., Yazaki, Y., Ikeda, M., and Nakao, K. (1968): Hemodynamics in juvenile hypertension with special reference to the response to propranolol. *Jpn. Circ. J.,* 32:981–987.
7. Levy, A. M., Tabakin, B. S., and Hanson, J. S. (1967): Hemodynamic responses to graded treadmill exercise in young untreated labile hypertensive patients. *Circulation,* 35:1063–1072.
8. Lundström, N. R. (1974): Clinical applications of echocardiography in infants and children. *Acta Paediatr. Scand.,* 243(Suppl.):11.
9. Payot, M., Bozio, A., Espelta-Vela, F., Fouron, J. C., and Davignon, A. (1975): L'echocardiographie: Une méthode d'investigation cardiovasculaire atraumatique indispensable en cardiologie pédiatrique. *Union Med. Can.,* 104:1642–1666.
10. Safar, M., Weiss, Y. A., Levenson, J. A., London, G. M., and Milliez, P. (1973): Hemodynamic study of 85 patients with borderline hypertension. *Am. J. Cardiol.,* 31:315–319.
11. Tourniaire, A., Blum, J., Tartulier, M., and Lestaevel, M. (1971): Hypertension artérielle labile. Variétés hémodynamiques. *Arch. Mal. Coeur,* 65:1179–1194.
12. Warembourg, H., Lekieffre, J., Bertrand, M. E., Ginestet, A., and Carre, A. (1973): L'hypertension artérielle labile. *Nouv. Presse Med.,* 2 and 22:1483–1486.

Juvenile Hypertension, edited by
M. I. New and L. S. Levine. Raven
Press, New York © 1977.

Clinical Pharmacology and Therapeutic Utilization of Antihypertensive Agents in Children

Bernard L. Mirkin and Alan Sinaiko

*Departments of Pediatrics and Pharmacology, Division of Clinical Pharmacology,
University of Minnesota, Health Sciences Center, Minneapolis, Minnesota 55455*

The proper clinical utilization of antihypertensive drugs requires both a clear understanding of their complex pharmacodynamic actions and a therapeutic philosophy that is consonant with current attitudes toward the value of intervention in the management of childhood hypertension. In this context, the therapist must be aware that some of the processes influencing the disposition of and reactivity to pharmacologic agents in the human (e.g., absorption, distribution, metabolism, and excretion) may be less well developed in children than in adults. As a consequence, any rational approach to the therapeutic management of such individuals must take into account how these interrelating factors may modify the clinical use of potent antihypertensive drugs.

THERAPEUTIC INTERVENTION IN CHILDHOOD HYPERTENSION

Selection of Patients for Treatment

Numerous studies of blood pressure frequency distribution curves have clearly shown that systemic blood pressure in children is lower than that in adults and does not attain adult levels until the second decade of life. Despite these observations, there continues to be a general reluctance to define hypertension during childhood on other than adult standards. As a result, considerable controversy surrounds the selection of a specific blood pressure, be it systolic or diastolic, which warrants the categorical diagnosis of clinical hypertension in the pediatric age group. Consensus of opinion appears to confirm the difficulty in establishing a precise cut-off for systolic blood pressure; therefore, children with persistent diastolic levels of 90 mm Hg or greater are considered to be hypertensive. However, selection of this level of blood pressure as the absolute upper limit of "normotension" for children may prove to be conservative when one views its similarity to the adult cut-off point in diagnosing hypertension.

Actuarial data compiled over the past 40 years by the insurance industry and population studies, such as the Framingham study, testify to the significant correlation between catastrophic cardiovascular events and incremental changes in diastolic blood pressure (1). Similar data in children are not available and the implications for children with diastolic blood pressures greater than 90 mm Hg, in terms of extended prognosis, have not been as well documented. It seems reasonable to assume, however, that the pathophysiologic processes attributable to the consequences of sustained hypertension in the adult are also initiated at the time blood pressure begins to rise during the childhood years. Furthermore, this view is consistent with data compiled in comprehensive antihypertensive therapeutic trials, such as those of the Veterans Administration Study (2), which suggest that morbid events occurring as secondary phenomena to hypertensive cardiovascular disease might be even more profoundly reduced if antihypertensive therapy were instituted shortly after the detection and confirmation of hypertension in childhood. Scientific support for this concept is available if one is willing to accept the spontaneously hypertensive rat model as representative of the human situation. Recent reports of greater longevity in spontaneously hypertensive rats given continuous antihypertensive therapy from birth suggest that early aggressive therapeutic intervention in individuals found to have elevated blood pressure during childhood might serve to alter the usual course of hypertension recently recognized to be a significant problem, even within the early decades of life (3).

It is surprising that the topic of antihypertensive therapy has not previously aroused a more significant dialogue within the discipline of pediatrics. A major aspect of pediatric health care delivery has historically been based on the principles of preventive medicine. The routine surveillance of blood pressure and initiation of therapy where appropriate might logically have been regarded as an integral aspect of pediatric responsibility. It is possible that the apathy of pediatricians in this regard can be attributed in some degree to the belated recognition of their colleagues in internal medicine that the increase of blood pressure in selected adults is not necessarily an appropriate response to the aging process. This misconception is currently undergoing extensive reevaluation among internists, although a considerable reluctance on the part of pediatricians to appropriately diagnose or initiate adequate therapy for hypertension still prevails.

Long-Term Consequences of Early Pharmacologic Intervention in Childhood

The cautious attitude expressed at the present time regarding the advisability and indications for antihypertensive therapy is founded on legitimate concerns. Serious questions concerning the consequences of prolonged administration of antihypertensive agents on the developing organism remain unresolved, despite more than 20 years of therapy with these agents in hypertensive children. In order to ensure that cognitive and behavioral development as well as somatic growth are not adversely affected, adequate longitudinal evaluation should be completed on sufficient numbers of individuals receiving antihypertensive medication for prolonged periods of time. Although some serious untoward pharmacologic effects have been described in children, they appear to be uncommon at present; the lack of relevant information serves to support a more prudent philosophy toward indiscriminate antihypertensive drug therapy. The caveat, however, is not to become a therapeutic nihilist, but is to develop stringent criteria for the appropriate use of such agents.

Problems related to antihypertensive drug therapy have been afforded only brief consideration in virtually all recent discussions relating to hypertension of childhood and adolescence. Energies have been directed primarily toward definition, identification, and evaluation of the hypertensive child, while provocative questions regarding therapy have remained unanswered. There are compelling reasons to develop a more complete understanding of the philosophic implications as well as biological effects of administering antihypertensive agents during the developmental years. If the current trend toward identification of greater numbers of children who require therapeutic intervention is borne out, it will be crucial to establish a body of knowledge defining appropriate dosing schedules, unanticipated consequences of prolonged drug administration, and accurate methods for monitoring compliance with prescribed drug regimens.

Assessment of Drug Therapy in Children

Objective information on the use of antihypertensive agents in children is generally inadequate and consistent with the prevailing deficit of information for most drugs in this age group. Approximately 85% of all the drugs currently prescribed for pediatric subjects have never been approved for use in subjects under 12 years of age or subjected to satisfactory clinical trials in this population (4,5). Dosing schedules have been constructed by extrapolation from adult standards and, although no overt hazards have been identified under these circumstances, one cannot but wonder what subtle changes in the developing child may be effected with extended use. Priorities and regulatory procedures must be established to permit investigation of these issues as an integral requirement in the design of standards for pediatric hypertensive care (6,7).

Establishing effective drug regimens for the pediatric patient is only the first step toward improving efficacy of therapy. As individuals within this age group begin to acquire greater independence from maternal influences, compliance becomes a major consideration in effective drug therapy. This is particularly true in conditions such as hypertension, in which the benign nature of the early course of the disease serves as negative reinforcement toward efforts to impress the patient with the potentially disabling consequences. Awareness of such a response makes it incumbent on the physician to ensure proper compliance. Appropriate monitoring of serum drug concentrations can be invaluable in facilitating adequate drug therapy, because experience has shown that the failure to attain an adequate clinical response can be related to failure to convince the patient of its importance to his well being.

CLINICAL PHARMACOLOGY OF ANTIHYPERTENSIVE AGENTS

General Principles

At the present time, there does not appear to be any single therapeutic agent that possesses the capacity for inducing a positive therapeutic response in all individuals. Thus, combined drug therapy is generally the rule in the management of hypertension, particularly that which is not categorized as essential in nature. As has been stated quite frequently, the etiologic basis for hypertension in the child differs markedly from that in the adult, with a rather high percentage being secondary in nature and a lower percentage falling into the category of essential hypertension. Despite the potentially greater possibility of obtaining a definitive diagnosis in subjects with childhood hypertension, even where the etiology is well defined, drug therapy must often be initiated in a manner similar to that used in subjects with hypertension of unknown cause. The main distinction between these clinical situations is that treatment in the presence of a defined pathophysiologic state may create therapeutic constraints. Conditions in which renal function is altered or where myocardial and vascular diseases co-exist may alter drug distribution and effector reactivity or cause some compounds to accumulate and produce untoward effects, unless the therapeutic regimen is modified to compensate for these situations.

Nearly all of the therapeutic agents currently available for the clinical management of hypertension in children modify the functions of one or more of the following: the adrenergic nervous, the renin–angiotensin, and the volume-regulating systems of the body. The most effective therapeutic regimens appear to be those which alter reactivity of these systems in the absence of side effects; these side effects can exert a pernicious influence on patient compliance and indeed make the "treatment worse than the disease." In this regard, therefore, it is quite apparent that the success of any therapeutic regimen depends to a great extent on the skill of the physician and his/her ability to exploit the many-faceted actions of the potent antihypertensive agents available for therapeutic use.

Since the commonly employed antihypertensive drugs have many overlapping characteristics, for ease of didactic presentation they have been arbitrarily categorized into groups that identify their major site(s) and mechanism(s) of action, as noted in the following section.

Agents Altering Electrolyte Balance and Fluid Homeostasis

Probably, the most commonly used drugs in the management of all forms of hypertension are the benzothiadiazide group of diuretics, commonly referred to as the thiazides. These compounds constitute the hub of most effective antihypertensive regimens and for poorly understood reasons can exert an additive, in some circumstances, even synergistic action when used in conjunction with other antihypertensive drugs. Although diuretic agents in this category—such as chlorthalidone and furosemide—differ in their molecular composition from the classical thiazide compounds [i.e., cholorothiazide and hydrochlorothiazide (HCTZ)], their effects on elevated blood pressure are quite similar.

Although the thiazide diuretics have been in use for over 20 years, there remains considerable uncertainty regarding how they specifically lower blood pressure. The initial effect of the thiazides is to reduce body weight by diminishing plasma and extracellular fluid volume via depletion of total body sodium (8). This is associated with a fall in systemic blood pressure caused by a decrease in cardiac output (9). Concurrent with these effects are hemodynamic changes which suggest a decrease in vascular responsiveness to catecholamines and angiotensin, and a reduction in cardiac output may occur, even before intravascular volume is changed by the diuretic effect of the thiazide. Thus, a direct effect on vascular smooth muscle and perhaps myocardial muscle has been postulated and demonstrated in experimental animals (10).

Despite continued administration of thiazide drugs, the plasma and extracellular fluid volume appear to return to normal, whereas peripheral resistance remains decreased below that of the control period. Recently, some studies have suggested that the patients receiving long-term diuretic therapy manifest a sustained reduction in plasma volume in contrast to the earlier studies cited above (11). At the present time, the action of thiazides in hypertensive states has not been clearly defined, except for the possibility that an effect of the drug, other than its diuretic action, must be operational.

The thiazides have been extremely effective in moderate and mildly hypertensive subjects in whom a reduction in blood pressure can be achieved and sustained during extended periods of drug therapy. In those situations where the antihypertensive response to thiazides alone is inadequate, continued administration of this drug is recommended in conjunction with other antihypertensive agents. This recommendation is based on data demonstrating that nearly all of the clinically employed antihypertensive agents tend to facilitate salt and water retention when given without a diuretic agent. This factor becomes rate limiting in restricting the effectiveness of these agents as blood pressure-lowering drugs.

The dose-response relationships in children have not been clearly established. However, a reduction in blood pressure may be frequently observed after 2 weeks of treatment with chlorothiazide (10 to 20 mg/kg) or HCTZ (1 to 2 mg/kg). Clinical studies have also indicated that no additional decrease in blood pressure or therapeutic benefit is derived by increasing total daily HCTZ dosages to amounts exceeding 100 to 200 mg (dependent on age and body mass). Loading, maintenance, and maximum dosage schedules for children are presented in Table 1 and are based on a consensus of clinical experience, rather than any detailed pharmacokinetic analysis.

Despite the widespread use of these compounds, surprisingly few data exist describing the dose–response relationships and elimination patterns of this compound in the adult; no data are available for children. One of the reasons for this apparent deficit has been the absence of microanalytical techniques possessing sufficient sensitivity and specificity to carry out these procedures. Within the past year, our laboratory and others have developed high-speed liquid chromatographic assays that are applicable for pharmacokinetic studies in young children (12). A typical liquid chromatogram is illustrated in Figs. 1 and 2, showing the pattern obtained when either serum (Fig. 1) or urine (Fig.

TABLE 1. *Pediatric dosage regimen for antihypertensive agents*

Drug	Daily starting dose (mg/kg)[a]	Dosage increment interval (days)[b]	Daily maximum dose[a]	
			mg/kg	Total
Diuretic agents				
Chlorothiazide	10	14	20	2 g
HCTZ	1	14	2	100 mg
Chlorthalidone	1	14	2	200 mg
Furosemide	0.5–1	14	2	—[c]
Spironolactone	1	14	2	200 mg
Vasodilator agents				
Hydralazine	1	3–4	5	200 mg
Minoxidil[d]	0.1–0.5	7	1–2	—[d]
Agents acting on adrenergic nervous system				
Methyldopa	10	7	40	2 g
Propranolol	1	3–6	—	—[c]
Guanethidine	0.2–0.5	12–14	1–2	—[c]

[a]Oral doses.

[b]The time required to achieve a maximum therapeutic response and/or steady-state blood level varies for each drug. Consequently, daily drug dosage should be increased over the time intervals noted in Table 1. Increments in dosage that are carried out over a shorter time-span may cause an exaggerated pharmacologic response.

[c]Maximal dose for these agents has not been established in children and is determined by therapeutic response or presence of adverse effects.

[d]Investigational drug available at present time only for use in subjects refractory to conventional antihypertensive therapy. Dosage regimen for children currently under study (Sinaiko and Mirkin, *unpublished observation*).

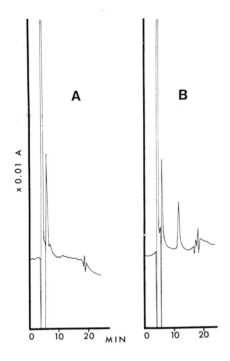

FIG. 1. High pressure liquid chromatogram of HCTZ. *Serum:* (**A**): blank; (**B**) 800 μg HCTZ added to blank.

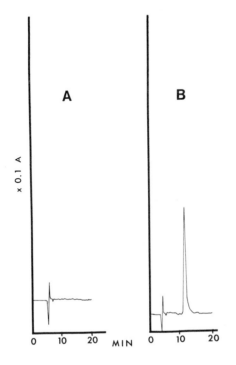

FIG. 2. High pressure liquid chromatogram of HCTZ. *Urine:* (**A**) blank; (**B**) 80 μg HCTZ added to blank. (Reproduced from Cooper et al., ref. 12, with permission.)

2) is subjected to analysis. The lower limit of detection with this assay is 50 ng/ml compared to spectrophotometric assays that have a threshold of 10 μg/ml and were formerly the only assays available. The serum half-life of HCTZ was studied in healthy adult volunteers, and a half-life of 5.2 ± 0.8 hr was obtained following administration of a single (1.0 mg/kg) oral dose (Fig. 3). These data are in agreement with those of other studies that were carried out in adults with the less specific techniques available 15 years ago (13,14). Studies on the uptake and elimination of HCTZ in children were initiated and a typical pattern is illustrated in Fig. 4. The peak plasma level following a single oral dose taken prior to breakfast was established about 2 hr after ingestion, and virtually all of the administered drug could be recovered from this patient within 24 hr. These data suggest that little if any of the thiazide was excreted as a metabolite in the urine. Considering the serum half-life of this drug, it seems reasonable to administer it no more frequently than every two half-lives (approximately every 12 hr) in order to maintain steady-state levels and optimum therapeutic response.

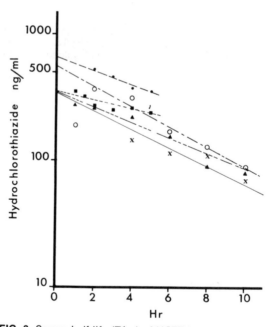

FIG. 3. Serum half-life (T^{1}/$_{2}$) of HCTZ in normal subjects.

Subject		T^{1}/$_{2}$ (hr)
1	(x————x)	4.4
2	(o— — —o)	3.7
3	(■--------■)	8.3
4	(●————●)	5.2
5	(▲————▲)	4.6

(Reproduced from Cooper et al., ref. 12, with permission.)

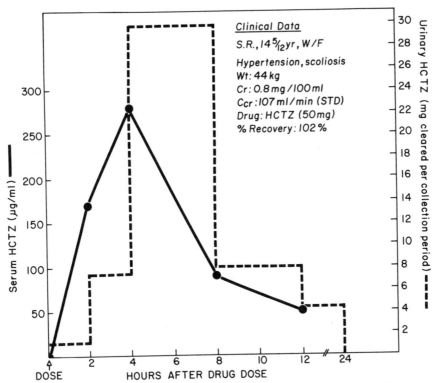

Clinical Data

S.R., 14 5/12 yr, W/F

Hypertension, scoliosis
Wt: 44 kg
Cr: 0.8 mg /100 ml
Ccr: 107 ml/min (STD)
Drug: HCTZ (50 mg)
% Recovery: 102 %

FIG. 4. Bioavailability and urinary clearance of orally administered HCTZ.

In view of the relatively rapid clearance of HCTZ noted in patients with normal renal function and the retarded clearance observed in subjects with decreased creatinine clearance, it has been suggested that an inverse relationship exists between serum drug levels and degree of renal function. A group of outpatients receiving HCTZ have recently been studied, and these data reveal a striking difference in patients whose creatinine clearance was below 50 to 60 ml/min as compared to those with higher clearances (Table 2). Peak steady-state serum levels of HCTZ ranged between 250 to 300 ng/ml in normal subjects, whereas those with impaired renal function had levels that were sometimes more than 20-fold greater. As a rule, HCTZ dosages are generally not reduced in renal insufficiency. It may be necessary to reevaluate dosage regimens in individuals with decreased clearances, because these high drug levels could lead to an increased incidence of adverse reactions.

The adverse effects associated with thiazide therapy have been well described for the adult population and are similar for the pediatric age group. Hypokalemia most commonly occurs during the early weeks of thiazide administration and can generally be corrected with oral potassium supplementation. This may create a major compliance problem in pediatric subjects

TABLE 2. Serum HCTZ concentration in random outpatient specimens

Patient	Diagnosis	Sex	Age (yr)	Wt. (kg)	HCTZ dose		Serum creatinine	Creatinine clearance	Serum concn. HCTZ (ng/ml)
					Total	mg/kg			
V. D.	Hypocomplementemic nephritis	F	12	45	100	2.2	0.6	118	125
R. W.	Turner's syndrome	F	15	52	100	1.9	0.9	117	197
F. G.	Nephrosis	M	13½	41	50	1.2	0.7	142	235
S. R.	Scoliosis hypertension	F	14½	44	50	1.1	0.8	107	280
M. M.	Systemic lupus	F	10	37	100	2.7	1.2	49	375
D. D.	Renal allograft rejection	F	25	45	100	2.2	1.3	—	540
A. G.	Oxalosis renal allograft	F	6	17	50	2.9	1.6	26	936
J. W.	Hypoplastic kidney	M	19	67	50	0.7	1.6	81	1,350
D. H.	Chronic glomerular nephritis	F	21	60	200	3.3	1.4	54	2,900
D. D.	Chronic glomerular nephritis	F	6	24	75	3.1	5.4	7	5,280

because the potassium salts are often unpalatable. Most children can be maintained in satisfactory electrolyte balance without potassium supplementation once equilibrium has been established, particularly if they and/or the parents are given adequate dietary instruction. Nonetheless, serum electrolytes should be monitored in pediatric subjects receiving thiazides because such periodic evaluation is essential for rational drug therapy. In circumstances in which potassium depletion cannot be controlled by diet, spironolactone is generally added to the regimen. This drug, while effective in most cases, substantially increases the cost of long-term therapy and the compound itself is not free from discomforting side effects. Spironolactone has been associated with changes in the periodicity of the menstrual cycle in young girls leading to emotional stress. In young males, gynecomastia is not uncommon and apparently results from the inhibitory effect of spironolactone on testosterone hydroxylation so that an actual decrease in this primary male hormone can be induced by the drug.

The incidence of hyperglycemia, hyperuricemia, or hypercalcemia in children taking thiazides has not been well documented but appears to be extremely rare in our pediatric hypertension clinic. It is important to consider, however, that extremely high blood levels of thiazide may develop in individuals with impaired renal function if the dosage is not adjusted, and that this may lead to an increased incidence of adverse effects.

Other oral diuretics have also been found to be effective in reducing systemic blood pressure. Chlorthalidone is a particularly useful agent because it has a much longer duration of action than chlorothiazide or HCTZ and can be given as a single daily dose. This is particularly valuable for preadolescent children in whom complex, multiple dosing schedules tend to create serious compliance problems.

The loop diuretics, such as furosemide and ethacrynic acid, are extremely potent and probably should be restricted for use in patients with hypertension and significant fluid retention not responsive to thiazide therapy. Hypocalcemia and hyponatremia may be produced by administration of these compounds but, unless severe losses occur, this is probably of less concern than hypokalemia. The degree of potassium loss can be so severe that potassium supplementation is generally required throughout the period of furosemide or ethacrynic acid usage, even in patients who have a marked decrease in renal clearance. Ototoxicity is a significant hazard and should be continuously assessed in subjects with impaired kidney function. There has been some tendency to utilize furosemide together with a thiazide for the specific purpose of reducing fluid volume in subjects who may not be sensitive to the less potent thiazides. This application is based on the premise that thiazide is a more effective antihypertensive agent. The rational basis for this combination still remains to be established, so that at the present time it should be considered as no more than a "clinical cocktail" of dubious value in patient management.

Spironolactone has been suggested as specific therapy for the treatment of "low-renin" forms of essential hypertension in the adult population. It has not been extensively utilized for this problem in pediatrics and a proper assessment of its efficacy in this regard cannot be presented at the present time.[1] There are several case reports indicating that spironolactone may significantly reduce elevated blood pressures in children with adrenal cortical hormone abnormalities. The aldosterone antagonists are especially useful as adjunctive antihypertensive therapy in those situations in which hyperaldosteronism may develop secondary to the nephrotic syndrome or congestive heart failure. Aside from its use in these specific situations and also perhaps to counteract the potassium-losing effect of thiazide diuretics, there appears to be no cogent reason why it should be used in place of the thiazides as a primary antihypertensive agent.

Agents Modifying Neurohumoral Regulation of Cardiovascular Function

Compounds modifying neurohumoral regulation of cardiovascular function exert their actions by altering some function of the peripheral or central adrenergic nervous system, resulting in a lowering of systemic blood pressure. These drugs tend to reduce vasoconstrictor tone and are most effective in the erect or sitting position when gravitational forces can exert a greater influence on hydrostatic pressure within the vascular bed. It is not surprising, therefore, to find that postural hypotension constitutes a major adverse side effect for most of these agents. Drugs that alter the activity of the adrenergic nervous system may act via a variety of different mechanisms and at different sites, as noted in the following section.

Drugs acting on the postganglionic adrenergic nerve terminal.

The major antihypertensive agents acting at the postganglionic nerve terminal are methyldopa, guanethidine, reserpine, and probably clonidine. Although this site may be considered the primary locus of action for these drugs, their mechanisms of action differ significantly. Methyldopa competitively antagonizes the conversion of dihydroxyphenylalanine (DOPA) to dopamine during the biosynthesis of norepinephrine in the nerve terminal. This results in formation of "false transmitter substances" that are less potent agonists than norepinephrine. Vasoconstrictor responses elicited by stimulation of the sympathetic nervous system are reduced in magnitude, which in turn leads to a smaller increment in net arteriolar resistance. Besides this peripheral site of action, recent studies suggest that methyldopa also exerts a major effect on the central vasomotor center, causing a further reduction of blood pressure (15).

---

[1]See New and Levine (this volume).

Sedation, the most frequently reported side effect of methyldopa, is a consequence of the drug's action on the central nervous system. It may occur shortly after therapy is initiated or any time during a clinical course when the dosage is increased. Methyldopa can accumulate in patients with renal insufficiency; if sedation becomes a prominent side effect in such individuals, the dosage should be decreased accordingly. Postural hypotension is also observed; however, most patients appear to accommodate to these side effects after several weeks at a constant dosage level. Other adverse reactions that have been reported (such as a lupus-like phenomenon and hepatitis) appear to be extremely rare in children, yet must always be looked for. A laboratory finding common in many patients is the presence of a positive direct Coombs' test which infrequently is associated with hemolytic anemia. If present as an isolated laboratory observation, a positive Coombs' test does not, in our opinion, constitute sufficient reason for cessation of drug therapy.

Therapeutically, methyldopa has been used mainly in children who are not adequately controlled with thiazide therapy alone. It is generally administered in an initial dose of 10 mg/kg/24 hr, given in divided doses every 12 hr. The serum half-life of this drug is approximately 12 hr in normal adults, and steady-state blood levels may be achieved after 5 half-lives or about 3 days of therapy. Consequently, the maximum clinical response to any given oral dose of this drug is generally not observed before approximately a week of therapy has elapsed. Increments in dosage probably should not be initiated more frequently than at 4- to 7-day intervals, with a maximum dosage not exceeding 40 mg/kg/24 hr (or 2 g/patient).[2] If a patient is still nonresponsive at this dosage level, the regimen is best supplemented with another antihypertensive drug, because administration of quantities in excess of 2 g daily rarely increases therapeutic efficacy and more commonly serves to intensify side effects. Particular emphasis must be placed again on the delayed clearance of this drug that can occur in subjects with renal insufficiency; therefore, a reduced dosage requirement and longer dosing interval should be considered.

Occasionally, methyldopa is administered intravenously when a more rapid onset of action is required. It is desirable to monitor dosage quite rigorously because rapid intravenous infusion of methyldopa in amounts equivalent to the daily oral dosage has been associated with irreversible coma in several patients with severe renal failure (Mirkin, *unpublished observations*). The cause remains unknown but possibly was due to the accumulation of high methyldopa concentrations in the central nervous system. It has recently been suggested that methyldopate (the ethylester of methyldopa used for intravenous administration) is not stoichiometrically converted to methyldopa in the body; therefore, it cannot be presumed to exert its antihypertensive effects via the same mechanism as methyldopa (16). Previous reports had indicated that

---

[2]The dosage limit for infants under 1 year of age has not been documented. It seems desirable not to exceed 20 mg/kg and to use longer dosing intervals, particularly in neonates.

methyldopate was completely hydrolyzed *in vivo* to methyldopa (17), yet only 29% of an infused dose of methyldopate could be accounted for as plasma methyldopa in the study cited. Presuming confirmation of these data, it is apparent that methyldopate cannot be equated with methyldopa, and this may be of clinical significance in view of the fact that methyldopate infusions have been associated with hypertensive crises in some patients (18).

Guanethidine is distinguished from reserpine and methyldopa in that it is selectively taken up by the nerve terminal and acts to inhibit the release of adrenergic neurotransmitter evoked by nerve stimulation. Thus, it produces an effect at the synapse that is analogous to the action of local anesthetic agents on the axon. Guanethidine is an effective drug, particularly during those periods of the day when the patient is upright and gravitational influences are maximal. By contrast, it produces a smaller decrease in blood pressure during the supine position and consequently is of limited value in the management of hypertension in neonates or infants. Another problem we have observed with this drug is that rather small increments in dosage can produce profound degrees of postural hypotension; therefore, a smooth regulation of blood pressure has been difficult to achieve in children.

Despite these deficiencies, guanethidine has some major attractions as an antihypertensive agent. Primary among these is its rather long serum half-life of 3 days, which permits use of a single daily dose to maintain steady-state blood levels. This has significant value when compliance is considered in the pediatric age population. However, the prolonged half-life also requires that a lengthy period of time be allowed in order to assess the effects of a given dosage regimen. With a serum half-life of 3 days, a period ranging between 9 to 15 days is generally required before the effects of any alteration in dosage can be adequately interpreted. In children, the maximum fall in blood pressure is often not manifest until about 10 to 12 days after initiating therapy. Thus, pharmacokinetic data, when integrated with biological response, may be of assistance in helping to devise more successful therapeutic regimens for individual patients, particularly for drugs that possess extremely long half-lives. In contrast to other drugs in this category (reserpine, methyldopa, and clonidine), guanethidine, because of its molecular configuration, does not readily enter the central nervous system, and sedation or depression are not frequently observed even after prolonged administration.

Reserpine, possibly the most venerable of current antihypertensive drugs, causes a decrease in the neurohormonal binding capacity of storage vesicles in the adrenergic nerve terminal. This agent has been used extensively in the past for the management of childhood hypertension, particularly that associated with acute glomerular nephritis. Because of the occurrence of annoying side effects, such as congestion of the mucous membranes, sedation, and exacerbation of emotional lability in preadolescent children, reserpine is currently rarely used as a primary antihypertensive agent in children.

Drugs acting as adrenergic blocking agents (alpha and beta).

Numerous investigations have demonstrated that the responses of the adrenergic nervous system are mediated primarily via the alpha- and beta-adrenoreceptors. Alpha-adrenergic blocking agents are seldom utilized in the long-term management of clinical hypertension, except under special circumstances where high levels of endogenous catecholamines may be present (e.g., pheochromocytoma or neuroblastoma). Within the past few years a large body of data has shown that stimulation of beta-adrenergic receptors (Types 1 and 2) can elicit physiologic responses such as tachycardia, bronchiolar muscle relaxation, vasodilation, and renin release from the kidney. As a consequence, many beta-adrenergic blocking agents, the prototype of which is propranolol, have been synthesized in an effort to develop drugs that will antagonize these responses.

Propranolol exerts its antihypertensive action by affecting the adrenergic nervous system in at least two distinct anatomical sites as has been previously suggested for methyldopa. Peripherally, it antagonizes the action of adrenergic neurotransmitter on beta-receptors and can suppress the release of renin from the kidney following stimulation of the renal sympathetic nerve fibers (19). However, the renal renin release mechanism can continue to be activated in the presence of propranolol under conditions that decrease intrarenal blood flow, such as may occur with renal artery stenosis or during allograft rejection reactions. Centrally, propranolol acts to suppress the intrinsic activity of the vasomotor center, leading to a decrease in vasomotor tone and a concurrent lowering of systemic blood pressure (20). Thus, propranolol may lower blood pressure in the absence of any effect on peripheral renin activity, and consequently suppression of plasma renin activity by beta-adrenergic blockade should not be considered its sole mechanism of action.

The pharmacologic serum half-life of propranolol in normal subjects is relatively short and depends on the route and duration of drug administration. In general, it rarely exceeds 6 hr and oral administration has been recommended at the termination of each half-life. The 6-hr dosage interval, although advisable for the general therapeutic use of this compound, is by no means a hard and fast rule because it may be possible to administer the drug over longer intervals and thereby achieve better patient compliance. No officially authorized dosage schedule has been presented for the use of propranolol in children; a starting dose ranging from 0.5 to 1.0 mg/kg/24 hr is satisfactory for children with hypertension. This drug is well tolerated in dosages and serum levels far exceeding those required to achieve a beta-blocking effect on myocardial and smooth muscle. Serum levels of propranolol above 100 ng/ml and dosages in excess of 1 mg/kg have been used in our clinic without any adverse effects noted in these patients (Table 3). In practice the maximal daily dose is determined by either the therapeutic response or the presence of any adverse effects. Children with a resting heart rate of 60 beats/min or less, or in

TABLE 3. *Relationship between propranolol dose, serum level, and plasma renin activity*

Patient	Date	Wt. (kg)	Daily propranolol Total (mg)	Daily propranolol (mg/kg)	Serum propranol concn. (ng/ml)	Plasma renin activity (ng/ml/hr)	BP	PR	Other drugs
Wanous, K.	5/4/75	20	20	2.0	8	9.4	138/85	78	HCTZ (100 mg)
Age: 6 yr	5/6/75	20	40	2.0	0	86.2	140/80	90	
Female	5/8/75	21	55	2.6	0	9.9	140/80	100	
Renal arterial	5/12/75	20	60	3.0	NS	22.8	140/80	100	
stenosis	5/20/75	20	60	3.0	58	9.4	140/70	80	
	5/27/75	20	60	3.0	240	9.7	138/85	78	
	6/3/75	20	60	3.0	NS	23.4	125/75	—	
	6/17/75	20	140	7.0	215	9.9	140/80	100	
	7/1/75	21	240	11.4	720	NS	130/90	92	
	8/12/75	21	240	11.4	300	11.1	128/82	88	
	9/9/75	21	240	11.4	NS	25.5	140/80	96	
	10/7/75	21	240	11.4	658	12.7	130/78	92	
	11/11/75	21	240	11.4	580	45.8	130/82	—	
	12/16/75	21	240	11.4	650	NS	130/82	84	
	1/13/76	21	240	11.4	590	22.7	135/90		
Anderson, J.	3/31/75	7.3	8	1.1	12	208	135/78	120	HCTZ (25 mg)
Age: 1 yr	4/11/75	6.5	8	1.2	90	122	178/70	120	Minox. (2 mg) + HCTZ
Female	5/27/75	7.7	0	0	0	60	150/85	120	HCTZ
Renal arterial	6/10/75	8.1	20	2.5	NS	21	130/90	104	HCTZ
stenosis	7/8/75	8.3	20	2.4	126	69.7	150/95	104	Minox. + HCTZ
	8/26/75	9.2	20	2.2	45	13.6	130/85	96	Minox. + HCTZ
	10/14/75	10.2	40	3.9	78	21.8	116/74	120	Minox. + HCTZ
	11/11/75	10.5	60	5.7	113	20.9	120/82	100	Minox. + HCTZ
	1/13/76	11.5	60	5.2		21.9	128/82	90	Minox. + HCTZ

BP, blood pressure; PR, pulse rate; NS, no sample.

whom the compensatory tachycardia accompanying the Valsalva movement has been blunted, may be physiologically compromised if increments in dosage beyond the current level are administered. Greater caution is required with younger infants and the resting heart rate should probably not be allowed to decrease below 85 to 90 beats/min.

The disposition of propranolol in the human is still under active investigation, but it does not appear to require any dosage modification in patients with renal insufficiency. These subjects have been reported to have a decreased serum half-life and to accumulate 4-hydroxypropranolol, a highly active metabolite of this drug (21). Recently, we have observed that extremely large quantities of propranolol and 4-hydroxypropranolol are present as the glucuronide in the plasma of patients undergoing renal hemodialysis (Mirkin et al., *unpublished data*). The pharmacologic activity of these metabolites has not been determined but is probably minimal and will be the subject of further investigation.

The use of propranolol is contraindicated in subjects with bronchial asthma or diabetes mellitus, and probably in those with a history of congestive heart failure. After widespread utilization of propranolol in the management of hypertension, this compound and its congeners have been officially approved by the Federal Drug Administration for such use. The compound has proven extremely useful in adult patients with essential hypertension in whom it appears to be both effective and safe. Similar documentation of its value in pediatric hypertensive states is not yet available, although preliminary reports suggest that this agent may also become an important adjunct to other therapeutic agents presently utilized in children (22).

Vasodilator drugs.

These agents diminish vascular tone and lower peripheral resistance by directly affecting vascular smooth muscle. The reduction in systemic blood pressure resulting from these actions is associated with a compensatory increase in the frequency of adrenergic neuron discharge and plasma renin activity as evidenced by elevations in heart rate, cardiac output, and renal tubular sodium reabsorption. Under some clinical circumstances, these reflex cardiovascular reactions may be detrimental and lead to episodes of angina, increased myocardial oxygen consumption, and occasionally myocardial infarcts. However, the concurrent use of beta-adrenergic blocking agents to blunt the compensatory physiologic responses of the body has greatly increased the usefulness of vasodilator drugs.

Hydralazine has been the major vasodilator agent used in the long-term management of adult hypertension and has also been employed in children for many years, yet it has never appeared to be as effective in this population as in that of adults with essential hypertension. A possible explanation for the apparent lack of efficacy in the pediatric age group is that hypertension in preadolescent subjects more commonly has a secondary cause and is generally more difficult to regulate than essential hypertension in adults. Recent data suggest that the incidence of "essential hypertension of childhood" may constitute a larger component of hypertensive subjects in this population than was heretofore thought to exist. Consequently, it appears worthwhile to reevaluate the role of vasodilator therapy in pediatric hypertension, particularly in conjunction with beta-blocking agents.

One of the major concerns regarding hydralazine has been its propensity for producing a lupus erythematosus (LE)-like phenomenon in children requiring high dosages, so that its administration to children with renal parenchymal diseases of immunologic origin creates a therapeutic dilemma. Oddly, the hydralazine-induced LE syndrome exerts a minimal effect on renal function, whereas other pathophysiologic alterations associated with the phenomenon are virtually indistinguishable from the naturally occurring disease. There are unfortunately no clear data defining whether or not preexisting immunologic disease states undergo exacerbation in the presence of hydralazine. Side effects such as headache, tachycardia, flushing, and nausea are also quite common, but they are significantly decreased if a beta-adrenergic blocker is administered in sufficient dosage.

A new and extremely potent vasodilator agent, minoxidil, is currently undergoing extensive clinical investigative trials. The antihypertensive potency of this compound is about 100 times greater than that of hydralazine on a milligram/milligram basis. It also possesses a much longer duration of action and in some patients receiving the drug, a distinct hypotensive effect can be noted for at least 24 hr (23,24). Minoxidil has a minimal direct effect on adrenergic neuroreceptor function and is similar to other vasodilator drugs, so that tachyphylaxis and postural hypotension are negligible. However, compensatory tachycardia, sodium accumulation, and fluid retention caused by increased sodium reabsorption in the proximal tubule may occur as with other vasodilator agents.

The therapeutic efficacy of minoxidil has recently been evaluated in children with hypertension refractory to other conventional antihypertensive regimens. This compound has been used on a short-term basis in patients with acute hypertensive reactions secondary to allograft rejection or progressive renal dysfunction, and in these circumstances it can produce a dramatic lowering of blood pressure with rather minor side effects (Table 4). A controlled therapeutic trial carried out in a group of hypertensive children assessed the efficacy of four different antihypertensive regimens in a randomized cross-over fashion over a period of 28 weeks (22). The regimens consisted of the following agents: HCTZ, HCTZ + methyldopa; HCTZ + propranolol; HCTZ + minoxidil + propranolol. The general conclusions reached from this study were that diastolic blood pressure was significantly reduced from con-

TABLE 4. Short-term use of minoxidil in the management of refractory childhood hypertension

Date		Antihypertensive therapy (total daily dose in milligrams)							BP	PR
	Diazox.	HCTZ	Furosem.	Spiron.	Methyldopa	Propran.	Hydral. (i.m.)	Minox.		
1/14/76	5 mg/kg	100	—	100	750	100	—	—	170/130	90
1/15/76	—	100	—	100	750	100	—	—	94/62	90
1/16/76	—	25	—	—	500	100	10	—	140/90	90
1/17/76	—	25	—	—	1,000	160	—	—	140/90	80
1/18/76	—	25	—	—	1,000	160	10	—	140/100	80
1/19/76	—	25	—	—	1,000	240	10	—	150/105	90
1/20/76	—	25	—	—	1,000	240	—	—	150/100	100
1/21/76	—	25	40	50	1,000	320	10	—	136/100	90
1/22/76	—	25	20	100	1,000	320	—	—	130/100	80
1/23/76	—	100	—	100	1,000	320	10	—	140/120	90
1/24/76	—	100	40	100	1,000	320	10	—	136/110	80
1/25/76	—	100	40	100	1,000	320	20	—	160/120	75
1/26/76	—	100	40	100	1,000	260	—	2.5	130/95	80
1/27/76	—	100	20	100	1,000	240	—	5.0	120/90	80
1/28/76	—	100	—	100	1,000	240	—	5.0	110/80	80
1/29/76	—	100	—	100	1,000	240	—	5.0	115/80	80
1/30/76	—	100	—	100	1,000	240	—	5.0	110/80	—

Clinical data: C. S., white male, age 13 yr. Renal transplant, August 1975; BP: 130 to 150/90 to 110 after transplant; diagnosis: stenosis of allograft anastomosis.

trol values (i.e., HCTZ) with each regimen studied, whereas the regimen of minoxidil + propranolol + HCTZ was the only one to significantly reduce systolic blood pressure below control levels. In addition, the minoxidil–propranolol–HCTZ combination also decreased diastolic blood pressures to a significantly greater extent than either HCTZ + propranolol or HCTZ + methyldopa; systolic blood pressures were not significantly different (22). A typical pattern of response in one of the patients studied is described in Fig. 5 (Sinaiko and Mirkin, *unpublished data*).

The major adverse effect noted with minoxidil therapy was the development of profound hypertrichosis in virtually all of the children (Fig. 6). This was not a dose-dependent phenomenon and did not constitute a deterrent to continued therapy in any of the patients. A similar response was observed in a previous study with guancydine and there were no overt endocrinologic abnormalities detected in either situation [Mirkin (report to FDA), *unpublished data*].

CLINICAL APPLICATION OF ANTIHYPERTENSIVE AGENTS

Pharmacotherapy for the treatment of chronically elevated blood pressure in children is best initiated by starting with relatively low doses of a given drug

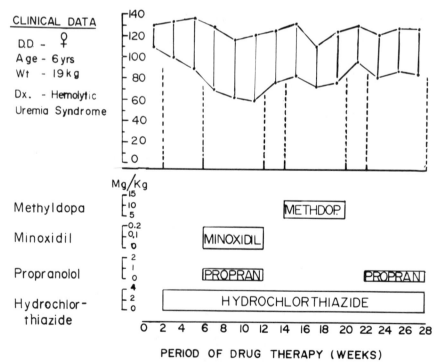

FIG. 5. Therapeutic response of patient in multiregimen cross-over antihypertensive study.

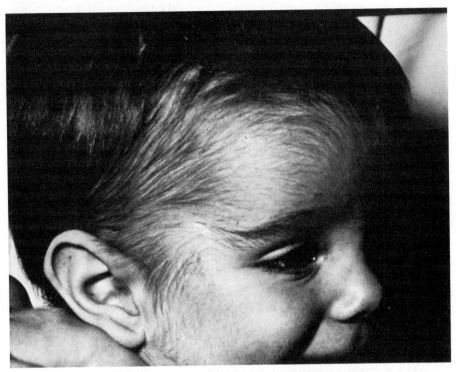

FIG. 6. Hypertrichosis in patient receiving minoxidil.

and building slowly to achieve therapeutically effective levels. This often allows the subject to accommodate to some of the unpleasant side effects of these drugs, such as urinary frequency, postural hypotension, sedation, altered bowel movement patterns, and tachycardia.

A large proportion of pediatric hypertensive subjects will respond merely to a decrease in vascular fluid volume brought about by diuretic therapy and/or sodium restriction, although the latter may be extremely difficult to implement as indicated previously. For this reason, oral diuretic agents, most commonly a form of thiazide, generally constitute the initial drug of choice. It is important to modify drug dosage according to the patient's renal function, because high concentrations may accumulate if this is not taken into account. If diuretics administered to the patient in adequate dosage and for a sufficient length of time evoke no clinical response, methyldopa can be added to the regimen. The actual selection of each antihypertensive agent is influenced somewhat by the pathogenesis of the hypertension and the age of the patient. Thus, in individuals with immunologically induced renal disease and secondary hypertension, the use of hydralazine or methyldopa, which both produce some immunologic side effects, should be carefully monitored. Infants who are generally in the supine position would be anticipated to exhibit a rather poor response with guanethidine in contrast to older children who are erect for longer periods of the day. In those circumstances where a child's blood pressure has remained elevated following the administration of thiazide and methyldopa, it has been our practice to convert the patient to a regimen consisting of a vasodilator agent in combination with a beta blocker and a thiazide diuretic.

Finally, it should be emphasized that all categories of antihypertensive agents, those causing direct vasodilation and those acting on components of the adrenergic nervous system, tend to cause some degree of fluid accumulation. Consequently, it is essential to administer a diuretic agent with all of the dosage regimens discussed.

ACKNOWLEDGMENTS

The preparation of this manuscript was supported in part by the "Program in Developmental and Pediatric Clinical Pharmacology"; USPHS Grant #08580, National Institutes of Child Health and Development.

REFERENCES

1. Lew, E. A. (1973): High blood pressure, other risk factors and longevity: The insurance viewpoint. *Am. J. Med.*, 55:281.
2. Veterans Administration Cooperative Study Group in Antihypertensive Agents (1970): Effect of treatment in morbidity in hypertension. II. *JAMA*, 213:1143.
3. Freis, E. D., and Ragan, D. (1975): Effect of treatment on longevity in spontaneously hypertensive rat. *Proc. Soc. Exp. Biol.*, 150:422.
4. Mirkin, B. L. (1975a): Drug therapy and the developing human: Who cares? *Clin. Res.*, 23:106.
5. Mirkin, B. L. (1975b): Impact of public policy on the development of drugs for pregnant women and children. *Clin. Res.*, 23:233.
6. Mirkin, B. L., Done, A. K., Christensen, S. N., Cohen, S., and Lockhart, J. (1975): Panel on pediatric drug trials. *Clin. Pharmacol. Ther.*, 18:657.
7. Mirkin, B. L. (1973): Research goals in developmental pharmacology. *Clin. Pharmacol. Ther.*, 14:762.
8. Conway, J., and Lauwers, P. (1960): Hemodynamic and hypotensive effects of long term therapy with chlorothiazide. *Circulation*, 21:21.
9. Dustan, H., Cumming, G., Corcoran, A., et al. (1959): A mechanism of chlorothiazide enhanced effectiveness of antihypertensive ganglioplegic drugs. *Circulation*, 19:360.
10. Frolich, E. D., Thurman, E., Pfeffer, M., et al. (1972): Altered vascular responsiveness: Initial hypotensive mechanism of thiazide diuretics, *Proc. Soc. Exp. Biol.*, 140:1190.
11. Tarazi, R., Dustan, H., and Frolich, E. (1970): Long term therapy in essential hypertension. *Circulation*, 41:709.
12. Cooper, M. J., Sinaiko, A. R., Anders, M. W., and Mirkin, B. L. (1976): High pressure liquid chromatographic analysis of hydrochlorothiazide in human serum and urine. *Anal. Chem.*, in press.
13. Moyer, J. Y., Fuchs, M., Irie, S., et al. (1959): Some observations on the pharmacology of hydrochlorothiazide. *Am. J. Cardiol.*, 3:113.
14. Anderson, K. V., Brettell, H. R., and Aikawa, J. (1961): C^{14}-labeled hydrochlorothiazide in human beings. *Arch. Intern. Med.*, 107:168.
15. Finch, L., and Haeusler, G. (1973): Further evidence for a central hypotensive action of α-methyldopa in both the rat and cat. *Br. J. Pharmacol.*, 47:217.

16. Walson, P. D., Marshall, K. S., Forsyth, R. P., et al. (1975): Metabolic disposition and cardiovascular effects of methyldopate in unanesthetized rhesus monkeys. *J. Pharmacol. Exp. Ther.*, 195:151.
17. Information noted in package insert for parenteral form of methyldopa (see loc. cit. 16).
18. Levine, R. J., and Strauch, B. S. (1966): Hypertensive responses to methyldopa. *N. Engl. J. Med.*, 275:946.
19. Michelakis, A., and McAllister, R. (1972): The effect of chronic adrenergic receptor blockade on plasma renin activity in man. *J. Clin. Endocrinol. Metab.*, 34:386.
20. Bravo, E., Tarazi, R. and Dustan, H. (1975): β-adrenergic blockade in diuretic-treated patients with essential hypertension. *N. Engl. J. Med.*, 292:66.
21. Thompson, F. D., Joekes, A. M., and Foulkes, D. M. (1972): Pharmacodynamics of propranolol in renal failure. *Br. Med. J.*, 2:434.
22. Sinaiko, A., and Mirkin, B. L. (1976): Clinical managment of hypertension with minoxidil: A controlled trial in children. *Pediatr. Res.*, 10:335.
23. Gottlieb, T., Katz, F., and Chidsey, C. (1972): Combined therapy with vasodilator drugs and beta-adrenergic blockade in hypertension. *Circulation*, 45:571.
24. Limas, C., and Freis, E. (1973): Minoxidil in severe hypertension with renal failure. *Am. J. Cardiol.*, 31:355.

Juvenile Hypertension, edited by
M. I. New and L. S. Levine. Raven
Press, New York © 1977.

Propranolol Efficacy in Adolescent Essential Hypertension

*,**Jean-Guy Mongeau, **Pierre Biron, and *Lourdes M. Pichardo

*Department of Pediatrics, Service of Nephrology, Sainte-Justine Hospital for
Children, Montreal, Quebec H3T 1C5; and **Department of Pharmacology,
University of Montreal, Montreal, Quebec H3C 3J7, Canada*

Essential hypertension is now recognized as beginning in adolescence, and the studies of Perera (5), Still and Cottom (6), Heyden et al. (3), and others have shown its long-term deleterious effects. A clear decision about when and how to treat these children, however, has not been reached.

Dustan and co-workers (1) have shown that after controlling the blood pressure of adults with hypertension for several years, 9 of 27 remained normotensive after the cessation of therapy.

In children, as pointed out by Kilcoyne (4), the fact that the course of hypertensive disease might actually be altered by early treatment has not been determined. The value of treatment in mild hypertension in adults, reported by Freis (2), encouraged us to study the efficacy of propranolol in adolescents with essential hypertension.

Our study does not pretend that propranolol is the only way, or even the best way, to treat labile hypertension; it was designed instead to investigate the effect of a beta-blocker in adolescents suffering from labile hypertension, hoping for a lasting, carry-over beneficial effect of the medication.

Ten subjects, five males and five females (14 to 17 years of age), met our criteria for essential hypertension, namely blood pressure readings repeatedly above the 90th percentile for their age and sex, normal renal function, normal rapid-sequence intravenous pyelogram, normal serum electrolytes, normal urinary vanillylmandelic acid, and at least one hypertensive parent. The term "labile hypertension" was defined as a blood pressure above the 90th percentile at three consecutive readings on different occasions, but the absolute value of this determination of blood pressure fluctuated from time to time. Patients were seen for 8 months by the same doctor, in the outpatient clinic, at

219

intervals of 2 weeks. Originally, six cases were randomly assigned to the propranolol–placebo sequence and six to the placebo–propranolol sequence. However, two defections for nonmedical reasons occurred in the first group and, therefore, only four patients assigned to the propranolol–placebo sequence are included here.

The patient was not aware of which medication he was given. Each sequence lasted 4 months. The dosage of propranolol was increased progressively until the blood pressure fell to normal value, and this dosage ranged from 90 to 240 mg/day. Three of these patients were obese (over the 90th percentile for age).

The results are expressed as the difference between the blood pressure of a child and the 90th percentile for his age and sex. The 90th percentile values were 131/80 for boys and 120/77 for girls. The mean values of the last four visits of each sequence were analyzed and the results of the systolic blood pressure are reported in Fig. 1. These results show that propranolol has an antihypertensive effect in all cases: the greater the initial systolic blood pressure, the greater the decline in the pressure. This correlation was significant ($p < 0.05$).

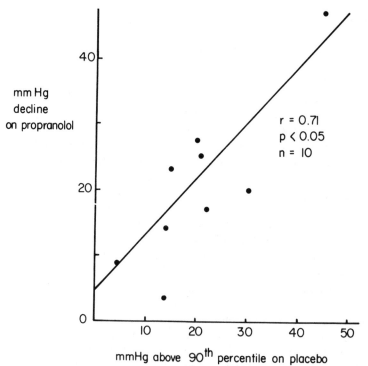

FIG. 1. Decline of systolic blood pressure after propranolol treatment according to the initial value on placebo.

The same effect of propranolol was observed on the diastolic blood pressure as shown in Fig. 2, and again, the correlation was significant (p value < 0.01).

These results seem to indicate that propranolol is an antihypertensive drug, but does not produce hypotension in adolescents.

Transient side effects were observed in three cases: fatigue upon strenuous exercise, bradycardia (45 beats/min), and a transient Raynaud phenomenon. None of these adverse reactions required cessation of therapy.

Plasma renin activity (measured with a radioimmunoassay angiotensin kit), normal in all cases at base line, was slightly but not significantly increased with propranolol ($p > 0.02$), which suggests that the medication was not acting via the renin-angiotensin system.

After cessation of propranolol treatment, blood pressure reverted to pre-treatment levels within a few weeks, indicating that there is no residual, carry-over effect after 4 months of continuous beta-blockade.

Hemodynamic studies were done on this group of patients by echocardiography. Detailed results are not available yet, but it is obvious that the effect of propranolol was better related to the initial blood pressure level than to the

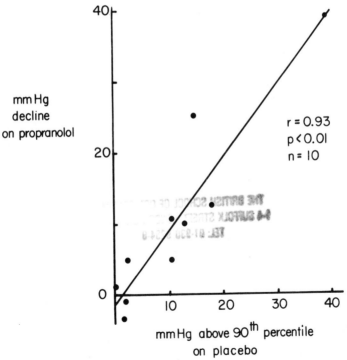

FIG. 2. Decline of diastolic blood pressure after propranolol treatment according to the initial value on placebo.

hemodynamic status; the hyperresistant normokinetic patients were often the most sensitive to the medication.

REFERENCES

1. Dustan, H. P., Page, I. H., and Tarazi, R. C. (1968): Arterial pressure responses to discontinuing antihypertensive drugs. *Circulation*, 37:370–379.
2. Freis, E. D. (1971): The chemotherapy of hypertension. *JAMA*, 218:1009–1014.
3. Heyden, S., Bartel, A. G., Hames, C. G., and Macdonough, J. R. (1969): Elevated blood pressure levels in adolescents. Evans County, Georgia seven-year follow-up of 30 patients and 30 controls. *JAMA*, 209:1683–1689.
4. Kilcoyne, M. (1974): Adolescent hypertension. II. Characteristics and response to treatment. *Circulation*, 50:1014–1019.
5. Perera, G. A. (1958): The course of primary hypertension in the young. *Ann. Intern. Med.*, 49:1348–1352.
6. Still, J. L., and Cottom, D. (1967): Severe hypertension in childhood. *Arch. Dis. Child.*, 42:34–39.

Subject Index

A

ACTH
  effect of unidentified adrenal
    steroid on, in juvenile
    hypertension, 143-163
  hypertension induced by, 69-78
  in juvenile hypertension, 179
  role in familial hypo-
    aldosteronism, 121
Actinomycin D, effect on
  aldosterone activity, 141
Adenomas
  adrenal, in children, 123
  aldosterone-producing, 171
Adolescents, *see also* Juvenile
  hypertension
  hypertension in, 1, 4, 25-35
    hemodynamic abnormalities,
      181-188
    labile type, 189-193
    propranolol therapy, 219-222
Adrenal gland, regeneration of,
  hypertension and, 57-59
Adrenal hormones, juvenile
  hypertension and, 7, 9
Adrenal hyperplasia
  mineralocorticoid replacement
    therapy in, 97-98
  salt-losing crises in, 101-102
Adrenal regeneration
  hypertension, in young rat,
    79-87
Adrenal steroid, unidentified,
  effect on juvenile
  hypertension, 143-163
Adrenergic blocking agents, as
  antihypertensives, 200,
  206-211
Adrenergic factors, in renin
  release, 89-93
Adrenocortical function, in
  genetic and experimental
  hypertension, 57-67
Aldactone, *see* Spironolactone
Aldomet, *see* Methyldopa
Aldosterone
  in children, 97-108
    plasma levels, 98-100

circadian rhythm in levels of,
  111-112
in experimental hypertension,
  58-65
increased secretion of, *see*
  Hyperaldosteronism
in juvenile hypertension, 9, 10,
  16, 37, 71, 165-167
metabolic clearance rate of,
  100-101, 106
receptors for, in kidney, 177
RNA synthesis induction by,
  141, 177
sodium depletion effects on,
  103-105
teratogenic hypertension from,
  84
unidentified ACTH-stimulable
  adrenal steroid and, 143-163
Aldosterone antagonists, as
  antihypertensives, 206
Alpha-blockers, as
  antihypertensives, 209, 211
American Indian children,
  hypertension in, 123-131
Aminoglutethimide, in low-renin
  hypertension therapy, 128-129
Androgen, hypertension induced
  by, 59-61
Anesthetics, effects on renin
  release, 89
Angiography, abdominal, in
  juvenile hypertension studies,
  7, 9
Angiotensin I, in juvenile
  hypertension, 30, 31
Animal models, for juvenile
  hypertension, 95
Antihypertensive drugs
  adrenergic blocking agents,
    209-211
  agents acting on postganglionic
    nerve terminals, 206-211
  clinical application of, 214-216
  justification for, 21, 23
  long-term use of, 196-198
  multiregimen of, 214
  neurohumoral regulators, 206
  pharmacologic and therapeutic